C000111527

BEYOND
THE
FAÇADE

By Eileen Chubb

'One million people commit suicide every year'
The World Health Organization

Eileen Chubb

Published by
Chipmunkapublishing
PO Box 6872
Brentwood
Essex CM13 1ZT
United Kingdom

http://www.chipmunkapublishing.com

Edited by Mary Dow and Danielle Atkins

Chipmunkapublishing gratefully acknowledges the support of Arts Council England.

FOREWORD

Eileen is one of the unsung heroines of our time. Years ago when I opened the first refuge in Chiswick, London in 1971, I was fighting to bring attention to the plight of victims of domestic violence. Nan was the oldest member of our community. She came to take refuge with us after a severe beating from her son. She died as a result of a frenzied attack from him when he was drunk. I was always aware of the level of abuse amongst the fragile elderly people in this country but the battle to even get the subject of domestic violence acknowledged amongst the powers that be in England meant that the plight of the elderly in this country slipped under the radar.

Whistleblowers anywhere in the world have to recognise that they will always be met with derision and abuse. We all grow up with the nursery story of the little boy who pointed to the Emperor with no clothes I always imagined his mother took him off and washed out his mouth with soap. As a nation the English do not like anyone who 'makes a fuss,' and I met Eileen when she was already cleaning lavatories to make a living after she was roundly condemned and blackballed by a major Nursing Home provider for daring to criticise their methods of caring for the fragile, elderly patients.

Eileen is an immensely courageous woman and this book is the story of her fight to gain recognition for the rights of the elderly community to be treated with respect and compassion. She tells the story of her brave and ferocious battle in such a way that the reader will be swept along and able to share her triumphs and the lows of what has become her life's mission. Her sense of humour never deserts her nor her archaic take on the pomposity of most of her enemies.

It is chilling in these pages to read about the lengths people in power are willing to go to stop Eileen and her supporters trying to protect their charges. That a woman of her integrity and compassion should be black balled from the caring profession and forced to clean for a living is a terrible indictment of our society.

I firmly believe that this book will reach a wide audience. All of us at one time or another will face the future care of our loved ones. Inevitably all of us will also look for caring as we reach an incapacitated old age. It is the Eileen's of this world who seek to make the changes needed and I am proud and honoured to write the forward for this book.

Erin Pizzey, Twickenham.

ACKNOWLEDGEMENTS

This book is dedicated to those I cared for during my time in Isard House.

I would like to thank those people who have supported me throughout this battle:

first my parents Nora and Patrick Chubb who never lived to see this book published, my partner Stephen Honour who is a real hero everyday and has supported me throughout, all those people who fight for the elderly every day, especially, Ruth Pool, Sue Sullis, Gillian Ward, Aureole Walters and Erin Pizzy, Gaynor Whitley.

I also remember those in the media who had the courage to stand up for the truth when the threat of libel deters so many from highlighting injustice: Heather Mills of Private Eye, Lucy Johnson, Sunday Express, Jenny Chyrss, BBC Radio Four Richard Simcox, New shopper

Finally I remember all those who have risked all to blow the whistle and do what is right. I ask the Government to do no less.

Eileen Chubb

PART ONE.   WITHIN ISARD HOUSE

PART TWO.   BEYOND ISARD HOUSE

PART THREE.   BEYOND THE FAÇADE

Eileen Chubb

Beyond The Facade

ONE

WITHIN ISARD HOUSE

I used to be very shy, people that know me as I am now do not believe me when I tell them this. I would never have complained about anything and had never fought for anything; it was other people who went on demonstrations and protested over injustices. In the past if someone had told me I would be demonstrating over the law's injustice, dressed as a judge in broad daylight in the middle of London, I would have thought they had taken leave of their senses.

I believe that we all have a limit, a line we will not cross and if we are pushed over that line, then our true capacity to fight is unleashed. Most of us will never be pushed that far. For those of us pushed far enough to fight back, it's simply because there are some things you have to fight for.

It's often the big things that creep up on us, the life changing events are rarely sought out. I did not wake up one morning and think "I will pick a fight with the Government or challenge the whole legal system." It all seemed perfectly ordinary when I look back.

I worked in retail management all my working life

and had reached a stage where sales targets were not the motivation they had once been; I was in a rut and wanted to do something different though I had no idea what exactly.

It was the summer of 1996 and, for the first time since leaving school, I did not have a job and I spent the whole summer sitting in the garden reading all those books I had always wanted to read but had never found the time to.
It was early autumn before I started thinking about a job and I still had no idea what I wanted to do. I thought I would flick through the yellow pages for some inspiration and I opened the book at random on a page listing care homes for the elderly.

I wondered if I should give it a go, after all my Mother had been a home carer with the local council for many years and she had absolutely loved the job, her "ladies" as she called her elderly clients, were like an extended family. I knew my mum got a lot of satisfaction from her job and maybe that was what I was looking for, job satisfaction. I decided I had nothing to lose by giving it a go, I rang the first care home and they offered me an immediate interview. I started work at Isard House a few days later.

I still remember that first shift like it was yesterday, I entered the building and was met by Val, a team leader who said she would show me around before taking me to the unit I would be working on that morning.

The first thing I remember was the smell, a mixture of urine and Dettol in equal parts. It was early morning so there were only a few residents up and about. Val explained as we walked that the home had sixty five residents in all and there were three separate units.

Unit one was the largest and had places for thirty physically frail residents, it was at the front of the building opposite the home's office.
Val said the other two unit's were for E.M.I residents. I asked what this meant and she said that before residents came into the home they were assessed and placed on a unit that suited their needs; either physically frail or elderly mentally infirm (E.M.I) which meant they had a form of dementia.

Unit two had seventeen residents with varying levels of dementia and was situated in the middle of the home.

Unit three had eighteen residents with severe dementia and was situated right at the back.

Val explained that each of the unit's had its own team leader and permanent staff team. There was also a separate kitchen, dining room and lounge on each of the unit's. She said Isard House was a residential home so there were no nurses on the premises, the district nurse came when needed and the G.P held a surgery once a week.

I remember thinking how big the home was as it had looked deceptively small from outside, I hurried along beside Val trying desperately to take everything in, when we arrived on unit three I was told I would be working there that morning as they were short of staff, but that I would be placed on a unit permanently in a day or two.

Val left me with a carer called Lizzie, who was in her late fifties and seemed to be very efficient despite looking a bit too red in the face.
Lizzie was very nice and put me at ease straight away, she said there should be three staff on duty but there was only me and her to get all the residents up, she said it was a shame I was being thrown in at the deep end and that she hoped it would not put me off.

Lizzie led me down a corridor on the left and said "This is Ivy's room." She explained quickly that Ivy was blind and wheelchair bound, "so you will have to wash and dress her." "I will be down the hall there if you need me", Lizzie said as she hurried off. I felt panic and realised I would just have to get on with it as best I could considering I did not have a clue what I was doing, so I knocked on the door and went in.

Beyond The Facade

Ivy was sitting up in bed, she was small and rosy cheeked with a mop of thick white hair which stuck out in all directions, "Hello Ivy", I said, "I am Eileen and I am going to help you get washed and dressed."

Ivy nodded briefly but did not speak, another wave of panic hit me when I thought about getting her out of the bed, I looked around the small room and saw a commode chair in one corner, which I brought over to the bed, I told Ivy I was going to slide her feet onto the floor and help her sit up and she gave the briefest of nods in response.

When Ivy was sitting on the edge of the bed I told her I would stand her up and turn slightly and sit her down on the commode, she nodded a response. I bent down and she put her arms around me and I prayed, please God don't let me drop her, and lifted her onto the commode.

I was so relieved to have got that bit over with that the rest seemed quite easy; I saw a towel and flannel on the side and ran some hot water into the sink, I told Ivy what I was doing as I went about washing her, I knew she couldn't see me so I thought she would feel safer if I told her what I was doing.

I went over to the wardrobe and found a selection of dresses and described them to Ivy who nodded her approval at a green one, so I got her dressed and tried to tame her wild hair but after a good deal of brushing it looked exactly the same.

I had seen some wheelchairs in a corridor nearby and told Ivy I was going to get one, I returned and helped Ivy into the wheelchair and opened the door to take her to the nearby dining room and I was just closing the door behind us when a loud high pitched voice startled me, "I like you I do, you're alright you are." I like you too I replied and I smiled and thought, "Wow what a great job this is", I knew without a doubt that I had found what I was looking for right at that moment.

Later on that day Sandra, the team leader, came in. I liked her straight away; she was wonderful with the residents who all loved her; it was a very happy unit; you could feel it in the atmosphere. I asked Sandra if I could stay on unit three permanently and she was very pleased as not many of the staff liked working on the dementia unit's. I could not understand why.
Sandra arranged this and I was placed on unit three from then on.

Over the next few weeks I got to know all the residents better including Ivy who turned out to be a real chatterbox and was just suspicious of strangers. I loved going to work and the more I got to know the residents the more I cared about them, they were just so incredible.

Isard House was owned by Bromley Council but

was contracted out to a company called Care
First, but it was sold to BUPA not long after I
started.

Lil was one of my favourite residents. She was
small and wiry with bright blue eyes that held a
hint of mischief.
Lil spoke with a broad Scottish accent and had
lived a hard life in the tenements of Glasgow.
Her mother had died when she was barely a
teenager and it had fallen on her to care for her
younger sisters and brothers. I think Lil had had to
grow up too quickly, too young and that's why she
was always up to mischief in her old age.

Just seeing Lil coming towards me was enough to
make me smile. I loved her for many reasons but
most of all I loved her for her innocence. Lil called
everyone "honey"and it rubbed off because I found
myself doing the same without even realising it.

As soon as she saw you Lil would say "Have you
got a cigarette Honey, I'm gasping for a smoke."
She was always on the look out for a cigarette.

She was just such a character and she had lived
in the home for quite some years so everyone
knew her. One of the other carers said Lil was
always escaping and one night she had got
several other residents up, put coats over their
nightgowns and taken them out with her. They
were missing for hours when the Police found
them miles away in Lewisham; how they had got

that far and had fish and chips and a fair amount of alcohol when they did not have a penny between them remained a mystery.

Lil had had to give up the escapades when she broke her hip and the Lil I knew walked with a Zimmer frame. When I say she walked with it, I mean when she got up to walk somewhere she would have to be told to bring her Zimmer. "Honey if I must "she would say and proceed to put it on her back like a rucksack, sighing that she was being made to carry such a burden when, as she put it, "I am no too steady on me feet and expected to carry this contraption Aroo tar boot."

Lil was always up to something and late one night I found her sitting on a coffee table cross legged like a wise little Buddha, watching the men's tennis highlights on T.V in the lounge in complete darkness. "What are you doing Lil?" I asked her, referring to her seating arrangement. She continued intently to watch the T.V for another moment as if to emphasise how unwelcome my interruption was before she turned her eyes towards me slowly and said in a tone you would usually reserve for a naughty three year old, "Honey I am watching the sport, there's a man with a rare backend on him there." I said I would come back later. "You do that now honey" she said her eyes already back on the T.V.

You always knew when Lil had been up to no good, a certain glint could be discerned in her bright blue eyes and the hint of a smile would appear at which point she would bite her lower lip to conceal it, but she never quite managed to do so.

I once laid all the tables in the dining room with cutlery and went to the kitchen to get china and on returning discovered every knife, fork and spoon had gone. I saw Lil half way up the corridor with her Zimmer on her back, a lampshade on her head and a borrowed handbag from which came a mysterious clanking noise swinging from her arm. "Lil", I cried, "I can hear you clanking from here." "Not me honey", she replied as she bit down on her lower lip.

Lil was in her mid nineties so every time she caught a cold or was unwell in anyway the G.P would be called out. I had not been there long so I did not know Lil had been consigned to her death bed quite a few times in the past.

I was working one late shift when the G.P was called out for Lil and, after examining her, had concluded it was unlikely she would last the night. I spent the rest of the shift trying desperately not to cry and succumbed to twenty minutes of sobbing in the toilet on my tea break. I returned to the unit and steeled myself to say goodbye to Lil and entered her room to find her bed empty and her no where to be seen. I went running to find Sandra and we searched the home. I found Lil in the hairdresser's room at the other end of the

building and ran to get her a wheelchair. After much cajoling Lil agreed to come back to bed, get in the wheelchair Lil and I will push you back I said. Lil looked at the wheelchair and then she looked at my red eyes and said in a very determined voice, "Honey I am noo getting in tha theng, you look in a worse a state than me, you get in and I'll push ye home now."
Needless to say Lil survived that night and many more besides.

Grace was a resident on unit three, she was tall, thin and angular, her warm brown eyes were the first thing you noticed about her.
Grace was a natural worrier and if you let her she tied herself in knots worrying about everything and everyone but herself. She loved a cup of tea but would only allow herself one once she was sure everyone else had had one first.

I would often find Grace in her bedroom, the entire contents of her wardrobe emptied out onto the bed and she would be sorting all her clothes into neat piles to give to the needy. The smallest of all these piles she intended for herself, "I have far too much, you must give these clothes to those with too little" she would say. Grace was one of the kindest, most generous spirited people that I have ever met, she would give you the clothes off her back without a second's hesitation, and she reminded me a lot of my own Mum.

When ever I got the chance I would sit with Grace

and we would have a cup of tea and she would show me her photograph albums. One photograph in particular has always stayed in my mind, it's of Grace as a young girl. She is wearing a long dark coat and one of those Modern Millie hats that come down over the ears, she is sitting on top of a long wooden gate and looking directly into the camera, a young girl without a care in the world just like any other.

Grace had a great sense of humour and she loved the parties we had on Sunday afternoons; on would go the Max Bygraves L.P and Grace would be the first one to start singing along.

She came out with the funniest things. Once I had been washing up and forgot to take off my yellow rubber gloves before going to clear more dirty dishes from the tables. I came to Grace's table and she shouted out, "Oh my gawd I thought it was a bunch of bananas coming to get me."

Grace would quite often refuse to go to bed and it did not take me long to work out why; she thought some of the others had gone out and would not be able to get back in so she had to stay up to open the door. I would tell her everyone was in bed safe and she would say "Thank gawd, I am so tired" and she would come to her room.

When I washed Grace she would say, "Fancy having to wash me" and I knew she felt embarrassed and I would say "You would wash me wouldn't you if I needed help?" Then she would smile and say "Gawd course I would."

I would bring her a cup of tea every morning and she would open her eyes and say, "Ooh a lovely cup of tea, have you had one though?" Her waking thought was always of others and when I put her to bed at night she always gave me a big hug and thanked me for everything.

I never once heard Grace complain about anything; if she was in pain, and she sometimes was, you would have to notice it for she would never tell you. "There is plenty worse off than me "was something she often said. I think that was an attitude you saw in Grace's generation, a kind of forbearance and strength to just get on with things. Grace had lost her Father and two Brothers in the First World War and she had two small children when her husband was posted as missing in action during the Second World War. He did eventually return home but Grace spent a long time not knowing if he was dead or alive; "There were plenty worse of than me."

The only time Grace would ever ask for anything was if she thought one of the other residents needed help and then she would come and ask the staff to help them.

You simply could not know Grace and fail to love

her. She was one of those rare people that made this world a better place by just being there. She spent her whole life doing little acts of kindness that enriched the lives of all those she came into contact with. I loved Grace most of all because of her generosity of spirit, she showed me what compassion really means and I will never forget her.

It was December 1996 and I had been working at the home for just over two months. I had got to know most of the staff and unit three was a very happy unit just as I had first thought. I really loved going to work and looked forward to seeing the residents.

We were getting ready for Christmas and decorating the unit; the Christmas tree was finished and we were hanging paper chains, which were a bit worn and tatty, in fact not a single one was intact; still it was beginning to look like a magical fairy grotto anyway. The residents were all watching the lounge being decorated and enjoying it, one or two would chip in from time to time with some advice as to where to hang a paper chain. An old Christmas LP was playing Bing Crosby's White Christmas, the lights on the Christmas tree sent out a warm glow that made the room look warm and cosy and all the residents were happy and alive.

Florie sat in the corner of the room, her bright blue eyes alert and taking in everything. She had advanced Parkinson's disease and her tiny body was totally rigid. She had not been able to speak for a long time, but her mouth constantly moved as if forming words that only she could hear. Suddenly her body would convulse violently and she would slide down the chair. Grace would always notice and find the staff to help her. When these convulsions passed Flories body would return to the constant tremor that rippled under her skin.

It was Flories eyes that drew you, they seemed huge in her tiny face, they told of her silent inner struggle with the cruel and relentless disease that racked her body day and night.

Florie loved to hear music, her head would nod and her eyes shine with approval; but what Florie loved most of all was to be in the middle of everything so she could watch all the comings and goings, as she watched the staff hanging the Christmas decorations. Florie was happy, her eyes, bright and alert, took in everything going on around her and for that short time she was released from the pain. She nodded her head and smiled as she listened to Bing Crosby.

We had a lovely time on the unit that Christmas, just seeing the residents enjoying everything was a buzz. I took photographs of them all sat down for lunch on Christmas day. We had pushed all the small dining tables together so everyone sat together. After lunch all the staff dressed up and did a music hall routine, I loved hearing them laugh and sing along.

Dot was a new resident on unit three, she was small and tubby with bright rosy cheeks and liked blue cardigans a great deal, and in fact all of Dot's clothes were blue.
She had only been in the home for about a week and spent her day on unit one, sitting in the large dining room, she only returned to unit three when it was time to get ready for bed. Julie, one of the carers, said that Dot hit her when she tried to get her ready for bed. In Julie's opinion Dot was extremely violent; I did not know if this was so as I had not attended to Dot as yet.

One evening I went to fetch Dot from unit one and I found her sitting alone at a dining table in a corner of the room. I told Dot that I had come to take her back to her room and help her get washed and into her nightdress. She was very reluctant to come with me but eventually after a great deal of persuasion and reassurance she came with me.
As soon as she stood up I could see she was absolutely soaked in urine and I wondered why the staff had not noticed this, but as Dot needed my full attention to coax her every step of the way I thought no more of it.

I had managed to get Dot back to unit three and was nearly at her bedroom when several other residents came out of the lounge with a carer. Dot seemed very startled by this and turned round to hit out and nearly lost her balance. I said "That's enough of that now" and we continued walking to her bedroom where I left her sitting in an armchair looking very cross. I said I would be right back and went out of the room.

I had seen something in Dot's eyes and wondered. I went to a nearby bathroom where on the wall there was one of the large Perspex containers that held rolls of hand towel. I removed the cover and placed it over my head like a visor and went back to Dot's room and knocked on the door and went in. "I hear I need to wear riot gear to get you ready for bed. Now do you kick as well as bite because I will need to go find some cricket pads as well" I said.

For a split second I thought I had misread her but then her face struggled to keep control, gave up the fight and she roared with laughter, the tears ran down her face and she fell back in her chair, she finally stopped laughing long enough to utter" Cricket pads" and then she was seized by a fresh bout, she laughed so much I thought she would never stop, when she finally looked like she would stop she would utter" Cricket pads" and start again. Her laughter was so infectious that I could not help laughing too. From that time on Dot and I were the best of friends.

Dot decided my name was Olive and that is what she called me. Dot was very shy really and when she had been taken to unit one and sat at the dining table for breakfast she had not known where to go when all the other residents finished their breakfast and left the table, so she just sat there. When she needed to use the toilet she did not know where to go or who to ask so she continued to sit there. She was sitting there without moving from seven thirty in the morning until eight o'clock in the evening and no body noticed she had been sitting there in soaking wet clothes too embarrassed and ashamed to let anyone else see.

I asked if Dot could stay on the unit and Sandra she said of course she could. I was made Dot's key worker which meant I was responsible for bathing her, as I could coax her to have a bath. She was not violent at all, only frightened and nervous someone would come into the room, so I would always make a big point of showing her the door was locked and she felt safe then. I told the other staff not to knock on the door as this always frightened Dot and it took ages to reassure her if that happened.

When I was not on duty all the unit staff were very good with Dot and did the same. Dot was really happy and well cared for, she settled in on unit three. That was why I loved the job so much; I watched Dot as she gained confidence, she was not the lonely frightened women sitting in a corner neglected but a happy smiling women who felt safe in her home. It cost nothing at all and gave me such a buzz.

Jessie and Rose shared a room. They were best friends, they had both been on unit three for some time and went everywhere together. They walked all over the home several times a day and Jessie would hold on to Rose's arm as they walked.

Both Jessie and Rose suffered from dementia. Jessie's dementia was much more advanced and she could no longer speak except for two words. If you talked to her for long enough Jessie would eventually say "Yes." The second word she could say was the word she used most; it was the first word she said when her eyes flickered open in the morning and the last thing she said at night; throughout the day you could hear Jessie say this word; it was the name of her dearest friend, Rose.

I realised Jessie was frightened the first time I tried to bath her. It was a Parker bath which had a door in the side and tilted back. I knew if I could just get Jessie to sit on the seat it would be alright after that, but Jessie would not sit. I knew that because her dementia was so advanced that I could not reach her to give reassurance with just words. I do not know where the idea came from but I started singing the song "Daisy", and as soon as I started to sing I saw Jessie visibly relax and I continued to sing as I gently sat her in the bath seat and slowly tilted the bath back.
I kept singing as I washed her and I was almost

finished and was beginning to get a sore throat, when suddenly Jessie sang out "You'll look sweet upon the seat of a bicycle made for two." I could hardly believe it all those words from Jessie, she continued to sing along as I got her dried and into her nightclothes. Once Jessie was sat next to Rose in the dining room having a milky drink, I was so excited that I ran all over the home telling the staff, some of whom probably thought I was mad, but all those who knew Jessie were amazed.

Jessie was never afraid to have a bath after that and no matter who was bathing her you could always hear the song "Daisy", issuing from the bathroom as two people sang it together.

Rose was Jessie's best friend, she was tall and broad and this was emphasised even more by her friend's slight frame. Seeing Rose and Jessie walk together you could understand why some of the staff called them little and large.

Rose was really friendly and called everyone mate, you could not help liking Rose. She was what was called the salt of the earth, she had a good heart and was very loving and caring, she would pause on her travels to greet you with "Alright mate?" as she passed you for the umpteenth time that day.

Iris was a new resident on unit three. She swore

like a trooper but had a heart of gold. I really liked her from day one. Iris always called me Doris, and one day I asked her son who Doris was and he said I was honoured by the name as Doris was his Mother's one and only friend.

Some of the night staff were afraid of Iris. I knew she would never hurt anyone. I thought because she swore such a lot they perhaps mistook this for aggression but that was just the way Iris had always spoken.

When I was on a late shift the first thing I always did was to go and say hello to all the residents in the lounge. Iris would be there and when she saw me she would give one of her rare smiles and follow me around constantly for the whole of the shift.

Staff handover would take place in a quiet corner of the unit; the morning staff would give an account of each resident to the staff coming on duty for the late shift. Iris always insisted on sitting with me during the handover and she would listen intently to each account of a resident, nodding her head wisely as if she knew who we were talking about and then she would chip in with her opinion of the resident in question, her comments usually consisting of "She's a right pain in the arse that one is."

Everywhere I went Iris followed and I always felt really bad when it was time for me to go home. I would take her into the lounge and settle her in a comfortable chair and tell her to wait there as I would not be long. She always said "I will come too" and I would reassure it was alright to wait there and have a rest. I would leave her sitting there while I went to get my bag and coat but I could never bring myself to leave without first checking that she had fallen asleep.

One day I was leaving to go home after an early shift. I took Iris into the lounge as usual and settled her into a chair and put her swollen feet up on a stool and told her to have a nice rest when she put her hand up to my face and said "Until the day I die I will never forget how kind you have always been to me." It was just so rare for Iris to show what she felt that it made it all the more special for her to say that to me. It was such moments that made the job so incredible and there were moments like that every single day.

Sandra, the team leader, always put the residents first and was always trying to think of some new activity they could do. She asked the home manager, Sandy, if she could have some money from the budget for pots and plants but Sandy refused. Sandra went and bought the pots and plants with her own money and a lot of the residents were able to have their own plants on the patio and they really enjoyed that. The unit was full of plants and fresh flowers. Relatives would bring in pot plants and they really thrived.

Edna was in her early nineties, which was really hard to believe looking at her, she walked so fast it was hard to keep up with her and I often found myself jogging beside her. Edna had been in the home quite a while and everyone knew and loved her.

Edna only ever asked for two things. The first was a cigarette after her meals. Sandra told me Edna's cigarettes were kept in the kitchen because she had kept losing them, so she always asked staff when she wanted one.
The second thing Edna asked, as soon as tea was over, was "Can I have a bath?"

Edna had no family. She had been admitted to a mental institution when she was twelve years old and she had been repeatedly sexually assaulted throughout her young life. Renee was one of the carers who had gone to see Edna in the institution and had brought her to Isard house.

Renee said it was heartbreaking to see Edna's reaction when she was shown her new bedroom. She had never had a room of her own in her life and slept in a dormitory with twenty other people. It explained a lot about Edna when Renee told me about her past. I would take clean towels into Edna's room and she would be sitting on the bed, she would immediately jump up and straighten the bedspread and I would reassure her that it was alright to sit on her bed. "It's your room Edna; you sit on the bed if you want to?" I would tell her and she would touch the bed and say "Yes, it's my bed" as if she could not quite believe it. We live in such a materialistic world and yet this poor women counted a room of her own to be such a blessing, it made you feel humble.

It was tragic to think what an awful life Edna had had and how very grateful she was for the smallest kindness. I think Edna was loved even more because of her past and everyone just wanted to make her last years as happy and safe as possible. Everyone felt it was the least they could do bearing in mind how her young life had been taken from her so brutally.

Edna was the most gentle person you could ever meet. I remember once I was walking past her as she stood in the corridor outside the kitchen door. She had her back to me so did not see me and as she turned round suddenly she knocked into my arm accidentally. She took hold of my hand immediately and started gently rubbing my arm saying over and over, "Sorry, Sorry, Sorry."

Florence C was a resident on unit three. She had been in the home some time, had advanced dementia and spent most days wandering about quietly talking and intently listening to herself. If you passed Florence on her travels and greeted her, she also smiled and said hello; it never occurred to Florence that anyone could be other than kind and she treated everyone accordingly.

Florence was tall and looked very fit; she had the body of a woman half her age. I suppose she had had to keep fit as she had competed in a man's world; she had been in the Auxiliary fire brigade. There was a photograph of Florence on her bedroom wall; she is the only women in a group of men, they are all standing beside an old fire engine looking very proud in their uniforms. It must have been very unusual for a woman to be in the fire service back then.

Florence was a gentle soul. She would smile at you while you washed and dressed her. Sometimes she would pat you affectionately on the top of the head in a distracted way as if she had just noticed you and then resume her conversation with herself.

Sometimes I would watch Florence as she talked, she would pause and listen intently and then carry on talking. I always wondered who she could hear but she seemed so very happy and contented that it really did not matter there was no one there.

Betty was a resident on unit three, she liked to help out with all the chores, she would lay the tables or help the staff put clean towels in the bedrooms, she liked to feel useful.

Beyond The Facade

One day Betty was helping with the towels when she suddenly stopped in front of a mirror in one of the bedrooms. "What happened to my face?" she said to her reflection." I must have slept on it funny for it to be all creased like that" she said to herself before moving on. I suppose Betty did not expect to see an old women staring at her when she looked in that mirror. Why should she? I never met an old person the whole time I worked in Isard House.

It was the spring of 1997 and I loved the job more then ever, it was really hard work both mentally and physically but the residents made it all worth while. A typical early shift started at 7am and there would be three staff on unit three to do the following tasks:

Eighteen totally dependent residents would have to be got up, washed and dressed and taken to the dining room.
Once all the residents were seated, the breakfast would be cooked and served and then we would feed those residents who were unable to feed them selves whilst we watched the other residents who were eating and prompted them to eat if they needed some encouragement.
We then did the early medication and then took all the residents to the lounge and seated them in comfortable chairs.
All the tables were cleared of dirty dishes and cutlery which was taken to the kitchen where we washed and dried up and put it away.

The kitchen was cleaned and the floor washed, clean tablecloths were put on the tables in the dining room and the tables then laid for lunch. All eighteen beds were then made, all the commodes washed and replaced, the clean laundry put away and clean towels and flannels put out ready for that night. And all by 11am. We then got to spend some time with the residents to meet their emotional needs in some way. Then all eighteen residents would have hot drinks. Several residents needed staff to hold the cup or they could not drink. Then all the cups were cleared, washed and put away, all eighteen residents taken to the toilet and taken to the dining room and seated for lunch by twelve thirty. Then the late shift would arrive so there was a chance to have a break. Then we'd return and, once the residents were cared for and comfortable, we would have all the care plans to write out before the handover of information to the afternoon staff. Late shifts were pretty much the same with bathing thrown in as well.

Jenny was a resident on unit three, she was from the north of England, she always reminded me of Agatha Christie's Miss Marple, she wore sensible tweeds and brown lace up shoes and looked very capable, she spoke in a no nonsense sort of way, she had wavy grey hair, warm brown eyes and always carried her handbag over her arm in the same way the Queen does.

Beyond The Facade

Jenny always liked to look tidy and she paid attention to detail. I knew she worried about the little things like if she had a clean handkerchief in her bag so I always made a point of checking before we left the room. She worried over whether she should take a cardigan and I would always say drape one over your shoulders and then you can take it off later if you like. They were such little things that it was no trouble to reassure her.

One morning I had hurt my wrist and it was bandaged and I was slowed down a bit and found it awkward serving breakfast and was struggling a bit. Jenny noticed and got up and came over to help me. I said she was really kind and thanked her. "It's not kind at all girl, its common sense, you with one hand and me with two" she replied briskly. That was just typical of Jenny, she always got straight to the point and told it like it was. It was the way she approached things, but it was only on the surface; underneath you could not want for a kinder person. She never failed to notice if I looked tired and she would come and give me a big hug as if she was giving a dose of medicine. "That will keep you going" she would say.

Jenny was the best of friends with another resident on unit three called Ellen, they had both come to live in the home around the same time, they looked after each other and sat together always, they were happy and settled in their home.

Eileen Chubb

Margaret was a full time care assistant on unit three. She was wonderful with all the residents who all really loved her. All of the staff on unit three were really sad when we were told Margaret was leaving for a much better paid job. I could not blame her for that as she had a mortgage to pay and I knew the wages were really bad. I was full time like Margaret so I knew she barely cleared four hundred pounds a month, so she left and the residents and staff all missed her.

Not long after Margaret left, the Deputy Manager of the home also left and she was replaced by a new lady called Maria Green. The management of the home sat in the office all day which was at the other end of the building so we rarely saw them, so it had no impact on us as such.

Some time later I was working a late shift and we were really short of staff. Maria Green came down to the unit and said a new lady who was a very experienced carer was due to start work in the next few days and that she had called her in early to help us put the residents to bed that night.

I met Maria Keenahan for the first time that night. She seemed very nice and I tried to make her feel welcome as was the way on unit three. It was small things I started to notice at first. There was something very wrong about Little Maria.

Beyond The Facade

As there were now two Maria's working in the home, the Deputy Manager, Maria Green, became known as Big Maria, and Maria Keenahan became known as Little Maria. Little Maria was placed on unit three permanently.

Margot was a resident on unit three and had lived in the home some time. She had advanced dementia and constantly walked around the home all day and all night too if you let her and did not remind her about her bed.

Margot had never married. Her life had been devoted to the children she taught as a teacher and later as headmistress of a large girl's school. Quite often pupils from the same school would come and visit her. They would walk beside her and keep her company during her constant travels around the home. I thought she must have been a very special teacher for her girls to visit her as often as they did. Margot received more Christmas cards than the rest of the home put together, cards from her girls all over the world.

Margot was a very genteel person and every person she passed by would be greeted with a very polite "Good Morning." I often wondered if Margot thought she was walking around her old school. She would stop often to look into a room and beam with approval at what she saw.

I had got to know Margot pretty well and I found

the ways to look after her in spite of her constant compulsion to walk. Her poor feet would be so swollen from her walking that they would hang over the sides of her shoes. I found a way to get her to rest. I knew she walked the home in circles so roughly knew how long it would take before she passed by the unit's kitchen again and I would have a cup of tea and biscuit's ready in one hand and just before she passed by I would step out in front of her and offer her my other arm and say "Shall we have tea? "She always replied "Oh how very lovely that would be" and she would take my arm and allow me to escort her to a comfortable armchair. I would sit her down and put her poor swollen feet on a stool and she would have her tea and biscuit's and promptly fall asleep.

I used this same method to get her to come with me to her bedroom at night but I knew I had to prepare the room first. I made sure the curtains were drawn as she became agitated if you tried to close them whilst she was there. I then made sure I had everything I needed to hand because if I had to go and get a towel she would be gone by the time I got back with it. In spite of having dozens of nightdresses I had to have a particular one, which was white with huge blue and red circles on it. If it was not back from the laundry I would go and fetch it. The story behind the nightdress was something I learned about Margot the first time I got her ready for bed. At least I had tried to get her ready for bed, but she became very agitated when I tried to help her undress and I knew it was

because she did not understand what was
happening to her and no matter how hard I tried I
could not reassure with words.

I picked up a nightdress and showed it to her and
she smiled in relief and quite happily let me
undress and wash her. That nightdress was the
same spotty one I used every night. It was the
only nightdress that worked, perhaps because it
was so lurid that she remembered it. It was not
really the kind of thing I thought Margot would take
to but because it worked that was all that
mattered. It took such a small thing to avoid so
much distress.

With all the residents there were lots of little things
that made them feel safe. It was just a question of
finding what worked best for each person. It is
these little things that help a resident feel they
have some control over what is happening to
them. When I offered Margot my arm I was inviting
her to come with me and when she chose to do so
she felt safe for exactly that reason.

It was by now the spring of 1997. Sandra's
husband was not very well and Sandy, the home
Manager, had not been very understanding about
it.

Sandra felt she had no other choice but to leave.
We all tried to convince her to stay but she did
hand in her notice and leave. I could not
understand why the Manager did not appreciate

such a good carer.
I will never forget Sandra. She is one of the
kindest people I have ever met, she taught me a
lot of things but most importantly that the residents
always come first no matter what. We all missed
her terribly.

When Sandra left, Little Maria was promoted to
unit three team leader in her place. It was not long
after this that the manager, Sandy, left and Big
Maria was made acting Manager until a
replacement could be found. Little Maria was very
pleased about this turn of events. She told me that
herself and Big Maria had worked together in
elderly care homes for over twenty years and had
always been the very best of friends. In fact it was
Big Maria who had got her this job she said.

Little Maria did seem very nice and she was
popular with all the staff. She was in her fifties,
small and dark with thinning hair which she always
wore in a bun. She always gave the impression of
competent efficiency. She was also highly
intelligent and completely charming. Little Maria
could recite, word by word, every guideline and
law that related to elderly care homes and what
was considered to be best practice.

As soon as Sandra left the whole atmosphere on
unit three changed. It was quite subtle at first,
nothing you could put your finger on exactly. I felt
uneasy and did not know why. I got on well with
Little Maria and I reassured myself that it was

bound to feel different with a new team leader at first. I thought "things will soon settle down again given a little time."

It started with little things. The first thing I noticed was that Little Maria never left the unit for her breaks. There was nothing wrong in this even though Sandra always insisted breaks be taken in the staff room as it made you a better carer to get away for a while. The next thing I noticed was the radio plays and music the residents liked were replaced by the TV which was now on constantly regardless of the residents.

The residents had always settled in the lounge before but now there was no music or radio they became restless and those who were able to move did so and wandered off; those like little Florie who were immobile had no choice but to stay put.

The lounge and dining room on unit three had always been the very heart of the unit. It was not just a big room full of furniture. It was home, a place the residents had always wanted to be. If it's possible for a place to die then that's what happened to unit three. It turned from a place where people once lived into a place where people waited to die, some prayed to die before it was over.

I asked Little Maria why she did not have her breaks in the staff room and she said she suffered from depression so did not like sitting alone. At first I had felt sorry for her and I thought she could not help it but my unease grew as time passed.

One late shift I was getting residents washed and changed into their nightdresses and I had gone to the unit kitchen to fetch some milk for a resident when I heard Little Maria shouting. I knew Maria was sitting in the front lounge, watching one of her soaps on the T.V. Grace must have got up and walked towards the door. Grace could not walk very fast and needed her Zimmer. I looked through the glass door that led to the dining room and saw grace at the lounge end of the room standing in front of the T.V. She was frozen to the spot in terror and sobbing. Maria who was shouting "Get out of my bloody way" was halfway across the room heading toward Grace and her face had changed beyond all recognition. It was no longer smiling and charming but contorted with rage and hatred. As she went towards Grace I knew she intended to hurt her and anyone who saw her face would have thought the same. My heart was pounding and I came along the corridor calling the name of a resident, I put my head around the door and asked as casually as I could if Maria had seen this resident; "Oh no dear I haven't" her face now completely normal and smiling. Grace let out a sob and I looked towards her; "What ever is the matter Grace?" I asked but before she could answer Maria said one of the residents from another unit had shouted at her. "I tried to comfort her but you know how confused she gets dear" she added in a matter of fact tone. I asked Grace if she wanted to come to her bedroom and get a cup of tea and when she agreed I said to Maria I may as well see to Grace as I can not find the other resident. Maria agreed and returned to her armchair. I do not know how I had managed to keep my voice light as I was shaking when I walked Grace to her bedroom.

Grace finally stopped crying and said "I am so selfish, people trying to watch a film and me walking in front of it." I told her it was not her fault and helped her get washed and into her nightdress and then said I would get us some tea. I went to the kitchen and turned on the kettle and as I waited for it to boil I had time to think for the first time. It suddenly struck me that I was in a terrible situation; "God, what am I going to do, report it to the acting Manager her best friend?" Just then Little Maria put her head around the door, "Is Grace alright dear?" "Oh yes" I said, she had forgotten all about it before we reached her bedroom and Maria seemed happy with my response and went off.
I got hardly any sleep that night and no matter how much I tossed and turned I could see no way out, there was no one in the home I could tell. The only other team leader I knew was Val, who had shown me around that first day, but she had left very suddenly after some kind of trouble with Big Maria.

Eileen Chubb

I knew it would be my word against Little Maria's and I knew who would be believed. I would have to leave and then what would happen to my residents? I decided I had no choice but to say nothing and watch Maria carefully, it was the only way I knew how to protect the residents.

Iris did not like Little Maria and when Iris did not like someone she did not have the skill or the inclination to hide it. Every time she saw Maria she would say "she's a nasty bitch that one." Maria did not like Iris and I was afraid Iris would become a target. Because Iris was still able to tell in spite of the dementia this gave her at least some protection compared with the other residents who were not able to tell.

I had noticed that Maria preferred attending to the residents with the most advanced dementia, residents like Jessie and Florie. I watched Maria constantly for anything out of the ordinary. What was the ordinary?
It was ordinary for day staff to work one of two shifts, either an early shift that started at seven am and finished at three thirty pm, or a late shift which started at twelve thirty pm and finished at nine pm. All full time staff worked a twenty three day shift pattern which consisted of seven days on duty followed by two days off, then ten days on duty and four days off.
Some of the staff worked double shifts or long days as they were called, but usually just before their days off.

Beyond The Facade

The job was so mentally and physically exhausting that a fourteen hour long day now and again with a day off to get over it would be ordinary.
The different shift patterns would mean you would attend to different residents on your unit, in fact it was expected that all the staff on each unit knew all the residents as you had attended to them all at some point in the last few shifts; that was ordinary.

Maria Keenahan never went home, she slept in a spare room above the office, she would get the same residents up each morning and put the same residents to bed each night, she was on unit three from seven in the morning until nine pm that night, every single day, week in and week out. Once she got her residents up in the morning she would mostly watch the T.V and if you asked her if she could help you make beds or with the cleaning, she would say she was not on duty. The only time she moved from her spot in front of the T.V was to take certain residents to the toilet. If anyone else tried to see to them she would say "That one is mine dear."

Time went by and still Little Maria had no idea that I suspected her and I knew this meant I was able to protect the residents. I felt really alone and wished that I could find someone to confide in but there was no one. Maria got used to me bursting into the room when she was alone with residents. I think she was really quite flattered that I needed her advice so much. I managed to come up with something to ask all the time, any excuse to get into the room.

I often found her gripping on to residents or restraining them, as soon as she saw me enter a bedroom she would smile and say she was trying to stop them falling.

I was due to have two weeks holiday in late August 1997 and as the time of this holiday approached I grew more and more worried. I think even Little Maria noticed this as she thought I just needed some reassurance which she gave me. "I will make sure the staff look after the residents dear" she said, thinking mistakenly that I was worried about any agency staff used for cover.

Not long before I was due off, I thought Iris didn't seem her usual self as she was very quiet. I remembered that her daughter in law had told me that Iris had always been prone to chest infections in the past and that she always seemed a bit quiet before the onset of an infection.

I went to find little Maria and asked her to come and look at Iris which she did and she said she was fine." You can not waste a doctor's time with old people who are going to die soon anyway dear "she said to me. I pleaded with her to call the doctor and she agreed to in the end, only because she feared I would not take my holiday.

Iris died a week later from a bad chest infection. She was seen by the G.P but it was too late and the infection had got too much of a grip. Maria had not wasted the doctor's time and had only called him out five days after I had asked, when it was just too late.

When I returned to work in early September Lil and Rose had also died and Grace and Dot were filthy and neglected. The horrors of unwashed red raw skin were to become all too familiar. I was at breaking point and then all the staff were told a new home Manager had been found and they would be starting work shortly. When I heard this I felt a glimmer of hope for the first time. It felt like the nightmare had gone on for ever by this point.

I could not stop thinking about Rose, Lil and Iris and when I had asked about their deaths I was told that they had all died of Bronchial Pneumonia and no one questioned their deaths. They were just accepted as due to natural causes and perhaps that was what happened. Little Maria said "These are old people dear and old people just die" but I could not shake the feeling that something was wrong, very wrong.

I kept thinking I had missed something, that some vital piece of information was staring me in the face and I thought if I went over everything I would see it. I was doing just that one early shift a few weeks later. I was alone and going from room to room making the beds when it suddenly dawned on me, the motive. It was how Maria's face had looked when I had seen Little Maria go for Grace. I had seen enough tired staff snap at residents in a moment of temper in the past but what I had seen in Maria's face was totally different, it was if she needed to inflict pain and she had been motivated by seeing Grace's fear. Maria had not lost control, she was never in more control and that was part of it. It had not been rage I had seen on her face. It was a lust for excitement. I felt a chill deep inside and felt physically sick.

The new Manager started work in October 1997, her name was Carole Jones, she was in her early forties, short and plump and seemed to be very efficient. I waited and hoped she would not get too friendly with the two Maria's. I had to report the abuse to someone and it had to be the right person if the abuse was to be stopped.

Little Maria was very manipulative with the staff, she would play one against the other and at first she had tried to involve me in the games she played, but she gave up when I refused to take the bait and react as she expected.

One of her favourite games was to target the younger staff. A lot of staff left and than I heard Little Maria telling a young carer that the other staff had complained about her. She said" I like you dear and thought you should know what is being said." Little Maria would always cover her back by making the staff feel they would get her in trouble if they said anything and that she was their only friend. Maria would then sit back and watch with great enjoyment the trouble this caused and this only added more to the already bad atmosphere on the unit and resentment and suspicion grew. Of course in doing this Maria drew attention away from herself and staff who may have witnessed some incident of abuse that troubled them do not tend to talk to each other if they do not know who to trust.

Another tactic used by Little Maria at regular intervals was to remind all the staff that she had the power. For example she would say how the home deputy Manager, Big Maria, was very pleased with her and how well she thought she ran the unit. "Big Maria just said to me yesterday that if any of the staff ever upset me they would be out the door" was something she told me more then once. These remarks were made in the most innocent way and delivered with the most charming, sweetly innocent smile, but the message that was intended was clear.

As soon as Carole Jones, the new Manager, started work, Little Maria made it known how impressed Carole was with her and how Big Maria had told Carole all about her excellent work running unit three. I noticed Little Maria would say things such as "I am just off to the office, Carole wants to thank me for doing some paperwork for her." What she was doing was making sure everyone knew she had control.

I think Little Maria had found these methods to be very effective in the past and they were effective because they made me hesitate to go to Carole Jones and report the abuse. "What if Carole did not believe me?" I thought, "It could backfire and then I might lose my job and the residents would be in an even worse position."

When you get someone up every morning and put them to bed every night for months on end you can not help but become emotionally attached to them. They are like a second family, which is hardly surprising as you spend more time with them than with your own family.

About a month or so later the team leader on unit one moved and Little Maria was very insistent that I apply for the vacant post of team leader. She kept on and on about it and she even went and got me an application form and stood over me while I filled it in. I went along with her as it never occurred to me I would get the job. I think Little Maria was desperate to get me off her unit because she could not control or manipulate me as she did the other staff. I also questioned her actions when no one else did.

I went for the job interview and can only remember one question, "What is the most important thing in this home?" I answered that the residents were the most important thing that no one or nothing came before them. I was absolutely stunned when I got the job and my first thought was for the residents on unit three, what would I do.

If a member of staff went to the office the whole home would know about it but if a team leader went to the office no one gave it a second thought as it was normal for team leaders to have a lot of contact with the Manager. I recalled the last home Manager, Sandy; from the time I started work up to the time Sandy left I saw her on the unit once and she never spoke and that was the extent of all contact. I decided that if I took the new job I would be able to judge if I could trust Carole Jones and the quicker I found that out then the quicker I could stop Little Maria, so I took the job.

I knew that I had a great deal to learn. Unit one was the largest unit with thirty residents who I needed to get to know and then there was all the paperwork that went with the job, time sheets, drug ordering, how to check the medication in and out of the home, the G.P reports and dealing with the G.P directly and then I would have to work two on-call shifts every week which meant starting work at two pm and working a normal late shift. Then with the added responsibility of running the home when the manager and office staff left at 5pm, I would have the keys to the office, would have to answer the telephone, deal with relatives and at the same time do all the normal tasks of a carer.

When the late shift finished at nine pm at night I would take a handover from the staff going off duty and handover to the night staff. Then I would go to the on-call room where I would spend the night ready to jump up if called to attend to any emergency, such as calling an ambulance for a resident if they became ill or had a fall. The task that I hated most was informing relatives if someone died. A normal on-shift would allow you two hours sleep if you were lucky and the next morning at seven am you worked a normal early shift on your unit, getting residents up, cooking breakfast, all the usual tasks. The Manager came in at 9pm and took back the keys, which was a relief as you did not then need to deal with answering the telephone which often rang just when you had a resident who was immobile half way out of bed. I finished my on-call shift at two pm, which was exactly twenty four hours later.

It took me months to adjust to being constantly deprived of sleep and by the spring of 1998 I had settled into the job and was considered to be a good team leader by the management. I loved the residents on unit one and felt a pride in the fact they were all so well cared for. I was exhausted most of the time because I still ran to find Maria and constantly interrupt her to ask her something about a team leader's duties, the usual excuses to interrupt her when she was alone with residents, only now I had to run the whole length of the home to do it and still find the time to care for the thirty residents on my own unit.

Ida was a resident on unit one. She had been the manager of a large office all her working life so she must have developed a stern look to go with her management position. Ida never married. I think her stern expression put men off which is a real pity because she had so much love to give.

She had thick grey hair that was cut in a neat bob, just as it was when she was twenty as the photograph on Ida's dressing table showed. Only the colour of her hair had changed, it was no longer dark brown but pure silver.

Ida could no longer walk and was confined to a wheelchair, she needed her hearing aid and it was the first thing I attended to when I went in to get her up. I remember the first time I got Ida up, washed and dressed her and she looked at me in her wise way and said "Yes I think you will do." It was as if I had just started work in her office.

That is what really mattered to me, that the residents were happy with the care they were given. It was behind closed doors so no one would know if you did your job well. Only the residents knew and when they gave their approval then as far as I was concerned there was no higher accolade. Buckingham Palace could give no honour or award to compare with this.

Eileen Chubb

Ida was wonderful but she liked to pretend to be stern and cross. Her act fooled no one willing to look a bit harder. Everyday I would come through the front door of the home and Ida was the first resident I would see in her armchair by the open door of the lounge. As soon as she saw me she would look around carefully and once she was sure no one else was looking she would give me a quick wave and a smile that was all the more dazzling because of its rarity. She would then look round carefully to check no one had witnessed her displaying such affection, and would then check the nails on her raised hand as if that would explain what she had been doing with it all along. No matter how tired or down I was when I came through that front door. Ida greeting me reminded me why the job was such a joy in spite of everyone that tried to make it otherwise. Ida reminded me how lucky I was to have a job with such rewards. "I haven't gone soft you know just because I gave you a hug" she would say. She always made me smile.

I was working an on-call shift when one of the night staff went sick and I took their place on the floor. I was really surprised when one of the other night staff said to me that Ida was very aggressive, I asked him to go into her room and show me how he normally attended to her when she needed the commode.

The carer nudged Ida awake and tried to get her

out of bed. She pushed him away and when he persisted she slapped him. He then said "See I told you she is aggressive." I said I was not surprised when he got her up like that; she cannot hear you firstly and secondly if someone tried to pull you out of bed in the middle of the night you would slap them too. He thought about this for a moment and then he said "It takes ages to adjust her hearing aide so I cannot tell her what I am doing." I said "Show her what you want." I went over to Ida who was by now in a mean temper which was hardly surprising.

I leant down in front of Ida so my face was level with hers and I could be sure her eyes followed my hands. I pointed to her and then I pointed to the commode and she nodded that she understood so I put my arms around her and she stood up and took her own weight and I turned slightly and lowered her down onto the commode. I did the reverse of this when I wanted her to get back into bed. The night carer stood and watched amazed and then said that he had no idea it could be that easy and had just thought Ida was aggressive. The carer had meant no harm, he was genuinely ignorant; "words are just one way to communicate" I told him. For the rest of that night shift that carer sought my advice on other residents who had been hitting him and after that he had no more trouble. I remember thinking that it took so little to make such a difference and it was a shame this carer had not been given any help before.

Doris was a resident on unit one, she was tall and slim and was one of those women who could still manage to look elegant even if they were dressed in a bin liner. There was this effortless grace in the way she moved and I thought she must have been a real head turner when she was younger. Doris had been married to a senior army officer and had travelled all over the world.

I was surprised that Doris was on unit one as it was obvious she was confused. I felt sorry for her, she got lost in the crowd on such a big unit and I always tried to give her a bit more time and attention whenever I could.

Doris spent her every waking hour trying to find someone to talk to, but because she was confused the words that came out of her mouth were not the same words as in her head and her desperation for company only made the problem worse. It was pitiful to watch this clever, interesting and witty woman desperately trying to find some friendship. The other residents did not know what she was saying so they said nothing when she spoke to them.

I would often find Doris walking the corridors sobbing her heart out "What have I done wrong, no one will speak to me" she would say.

Beyond The Facade

I would take her with me and get her a drink and then sit down with her listening and reassuring her. Once she relaxed the right words often came naturally, it was such a pity. Doris was locked into this world of silence and isolation and it was a living hell for this clever genteel women who craved human contact above all else.

Ethel was a resident on unit one, she was big and round and extremely jolly, she did look quite ladylike but she very soon shattered that illusion when she recited tales of her younger days. "I was a right goer I was you know" was her favourite expression.

The more shock she saw on the face of her listener, the more Ethel roared with laughter. You could actually see the staff all tense when a Vicar or Priest walked through the door. Ethel would have seen him first and would already be making a beeline for them, a wicked grin of anticipation of her face.

I remember one late shift in particular, all the residents were in the lounge and I was taking the tea trolley around the large room and I had just stopped in front of Ethel when a male resident who was walking across the room suddenly found his trousers had fallen down around his ankles. There was a loud gasp as twenty elderly ladies put their hands over their eyes. Not Ethel though. She was not content with a discreet peep, she stood up and said to me very loudly, "Oh do get out of the way duck, you are blocking my view" and that was pretty much typical Ethel.

Lizzie was a new resident on unit one, she was tiny and looked like a little pixie, she came from the west of Ireland originally and in spite of having lived in England for over thirty years, she still spoke with a very broad Irish accent.

I met Lizzie for the first time one morning when I went to her bedroom to help her get washed and dressed. I was expecting to find a physically frail resident but I was greeted by this robust little woman whose first words to me were, "Jesus, there is a big bee at the window there and he's after telling everyone I slept with the British Government and I never did now." I was taken aback at first, not by the bee thing but because Lizzie was on a physically frail unit when she was obviously confused.

Every resident is different, that I knew and I had learnt that different things worked when it came to dealing with dementia.
When it came to residents who were as distressed as Lizzie was over the bee, you could go down two roads; either deny that the bee was there and give plenty of reassurance that there never was a bee and that it was all a huge mistake, or accept that the bee was there but reason that what it was saying was wrong. I quickly judged the later approach might work better for Lizzie so I said

Beyond The Facade

"Now whose going to believe that bee? Who would sleep with that ugly lot?" Lizzie immediately relaxed and soon forgot all about the bee.

I really liked Lizzie, she was a lovely lady and she had worried all her life but now the dementia meant her worries took all shapes and forms and I knew she needed someone who would just listen to her fears and make sense of the crazy things going on around her.

What ever was going on she always remembered my name and as soon as she saw me would call "Eileen, Eileen, quick come here now." I would ask her what was wrong "There's been a terrible to do while you were out and the police and all were after coming and they took that man over there, he's only after stealing all the chairs now he is." Lizzie would then look at me expectantly waiting for me to explain it all to her and make it alright. I really do not know how I came up with the answers but I always managed to think of something to reassure her and this time I told her the man was moving furniture and had just gone to the wrong house.

Whatever you have to do to make a resident feel safe you just do it, no matter how crazy or far fetched it seems to you, to that person it's real and so is the distress they feel, there is always a way to help people like Lizzie if you really want to. When ever I came up with the answer Lizzie would relax back into her chair and for a while she felt safe. She always said to me "Jasus it's bedlam in this place the minute you go out of that door."

I ran down to unit three when ever I could, it was nearly Christmas 1997, what a difference a year makes.

I remembered last Christmas on unit three, hanging the decorations, the happy animated faces of the residents, Bing Crosby singing White Christmas and how cosy the room looked in the glow of the lights on the tree. God was it really only this time last year, I thought, the memories seemed so much more vivid compared to the scene that now greeted me,
 A few bit's of tinsel which had been half-heartedly draped here and there, the rest of the decorations and the Christmas tree were absent, they had been placed in the back lounge which had become an unofficial staff room and was where Little Maria now sat watching T.V. The residents were left to sit alone in the front lounge, alone and in deathly silence. The room seemed so much darker somehow and the residents were either asleep or staring into space in a dazed stupor, even all the plants had died, their brittle brown leaves left where they fell, a bitter reminder that life had once flourished in those withered remains.

The months passed and I learnt about the medication system and as my knowledge grew so did my suspicions. I saw Margot wandering, she looked so much thinner and her skin showed the signs of dehydration. I started to look out for her at mealtimes, sometimes I caught sight of her as she walked in her never ending circles or if I missed her I would save some of the food and a drink for her to have later.

Poor Margot, she was so pitifully grateful when she saw the food I held out and she would thank me profusely. She had always been such a ladylike person, especially her table manners, she always ate so daintily but now she crammed the food into her mouth and she would gulp down four or five cups of tea as if her life depended on it, which of course it did.

Then the night staff who had been there for years started to complain. They said they were being blamed for the cuts, bruises and black eyes that were occurring on unit three. It was the summer of 1998. I was due to have two weeks holiday, the day before I went on leave Carole Jones said she was going to rotate all the team leaders. Little Maria was placed on unit two, Amanda, a new team leader, was placed on unit one and I was placed on unit three. Nothing that I had seen or suspected or even imagined in my worst nightmare could have prepared me for what I was about to find.

I returned from my two weeks holiday to work my first shift as unit three team leader.

Eileen Chubb

Jessie was the first resident I went to get up that morning. I went to her room and sat her up in bed which was difficult as she flinched from all contact so I did the only thing I could think of and that was to sing to her. I sang, "Daisy"and after I had sung a while she relaxed and then faltering she stumbled over the words of the first verse and looked at me and said "Rose?" As if it were a question she was asking. I kept on singing and removed her nightdress, there were finger mark bruises up both her arms, her back was covered in a mixture of yellow, green and black bruises and when I removed her incontinence pad she cried out "Rose" in an expression of pain. There were urine burns, the most recent of which were red raw and covered in weeping blisters; brown, puckered, thick scar tissue showed where earlier burns had been inflicted. I gently washed Jessie and covered her burns in barrier cream and I sang to her as I did this and it was the salt in my mouth that made me realise there tears were streaming down my face.

I kept going on some kind of automatic pilot, on to the next resident. The next fold of skin lifted, the rancid stench of another sweat rash oozing blisters in festering folds of long unwashed skin, kept permanently damp by pus and sweat, more urine burns red raw blistered skin, more dehydrated bruised bodies lying on filthy sheets soaked in urine or stiff with blood and pus.

Beyond The Facade

When I knocked and entered Grace's room she
had her hands over her head and cried out
"Please don't hurt me." That kind of broke the spell
and I snapped awake, the silent tears now
reached my throat and I swallowed hard to
suppress the sob that threatened to overcome me.
I felt the first stirring of anger then and had Carole
Jones been in the home right then I would have
run and got her but she was away for a couple of
days and my heart sank at the thought of having
to wait. God I thought I will have to avoid Maria
because if I had seen her I would have been more
then tempted to knock her down where she stood
and that is the only time in my life that I was
tempted to use violence.

I knew I had to keep myself together and when
Little Maria walked on to the unit later that morning
I held my breath and dug my nails into my palm.
"Big Maria wants to know if any staff on this unit
have been telling tales about me as she will have
them out." I looked at her and knew it was a clear
threat but I struggled for control and said nothing.
She sat there on unit three that morning silently
watching everything and I asked her why she said
she was not on duty.

Renee was one of the other carers, she had
worked on unit three before and had recently
moved back onto the unit. She heard me asking
Maria why she was on unit three and she came
and told me later that Little Maria had spent all her
time on unit three when I was on holiday and had

not worked on her own unit at all.

I counted the hours until Carole Jones returned and while I waited every shift brought fresh discoveries of abuse.
The medication trolley was stuffed with illegally stockpiled medication, residents discontinued medication was not returned and neither had the medication of residents who had died been sent back. There were controlled drugs everywhere, drugs were recorded as given to residents that were not prescribed to them, there was overdosing and drugs withheld. I just felt overwhelmed by the sheer scale of it.

The morning that Carole Jones returned I went to the office and asked if I could speak to her urgently and that I wanted Little Maria to be present as what I had to say concerned her. I think Carole could see how urgent it was from the look on my face and shortly after all three of us were seated in the conference room upstairs. I opened my mouth and it all poured out, what I had seen before and all the abuse I had discovered since. Maria tried to drown me out but gave up. I had waited to speak for too long to be silenced now and I told about the threats that were used to keep everyone silent, why I had waited to speak to her and finally about Little Maria being on my unit when her own unit had no staff and that I may as well go and work on unit two. This last bit was only to emphasise that unit two had no team leader, I was most certainly not expecting Carole to say that I should go to unit two and Little Maria should return to unit three. I left the room knowing I had risked all and failed. Little Maria followed me and said "Your Dot will pay for this."

I returned to unit three to get my bag and coat. Renee was in the kitchen and asked me why I was going. I said I had no choice and could say nothing else about it.
I walked around to unit two with a heavy heart and I saw a member of staff in the hallway and asked what help they needed, the carer looked a bit puzzled as to why I was on the unit but she did not ask any questions and said the beds had yet to be made. I went and got clean linen and made my way to the first of the bedrooms, I was grateful for some time alone to think things over. I realised that I was now in the position that I had always dreaded; both of the Maria's knew I was a real threat to them and they both had the power to make my working life hell. I felt really vulnerable and thought it was only a matter of time before I would be forced out.

I continued making the beds and had reached the third or fourth bedroom when I heard someone knocking at the doors a little way down the corridor. I looked out into the hallway and saw Carole Jones, she said she had been looking for me and that we needed to talk, she came into the bedroom and closed the door. She told me that she knew what I had said earlier was true and had suspected something was wrong for a while. She

said she could sack Maria Keenahan immediately but she could go and get a job in another care home and abuse more residents in future and surely I would not want that. She then went on to say that if I helped her to collect enough evidence against Maria then she could ensure she never worked in care again. This seemed reasonable to me. "But what about the residents, will they be safe? "I asked her and she assured they would be in no danger and that she had moved little Maria back to unit three only to give her enough rope to hang herself, then it would not take long to gather all the evidence that was needed and once Little Maria went her friend big Maria would not stay.
I was so relieved at last not to have to carry the burden on my own that I believed this and I trusted Carole Jones to act. It honestly never occurred to me to question this. Just before she left the room Carole said I was not to speak of this matter to any one else under any circumstances and I gave her my word I would not and she left. I carried on making the beds but now I felt there was hope at last and trusted that Carole would not let the two Maria's do anything to harm any more residents or to make my working life hard now she knew about the abuse.

Little Maria told all the staff that Carole had moved her back to unit three because unit two made her feel claustrophobic. Perhaps it did make her feel hemmed in and her excuse had some truth in it, after all Little Maria did not like being over looked and unit two being in the centre of the home was more over looked than the other unit's, and unit three was the least looked over and the back lounge on unit three was the most secret place of all.

Since the night of the Grace incident, I had watched Little Maria closely and given a great deal of thought to what made her tick. I knew Maria needed to abuse because it made her feel powerful and that power was her fix. She needed it to exist and that's why she lived in the home, it gave her access to her victims around the clock.

Little Maria was an excellent actress and could play the part of stupid, ignorant or concerned carer with ease. She could also switch from one part to another if she felt it would be more effective. She had once boasted that Big Maria always let her deal with awkward relatives, "You know the ones that are always moaning" she said and I could see why Big Maria made use of such skills as Little Maria had an answer for everything. I watched her charm and sow doubt in the mind of concerned relatives many times, by the time she had finished with them it was the relative who felt they were being unreasonable.

Little Maria manipulated staff for the same reason; it suited her purpose. The good staff on unit three eventually all left the home or moved to other unit's. Maria then attracted to her other staff who abused and her inner circle on unit three shortly became a circle of abusers. The only other staff she would tolerate on the unit were young inexperienced carers who could easily be controlled. Lee and Lizzy were two such young carers and they were excellent with the residents so it was not long before Maria began to view them as a threat to be dealt with. This manipulation and control of the staff was all part of the excitement for Little Maria, they were challenges she had to overcome in order to abuse and were part of the game to her.

Jackie worked on unit three as a care assistant, she had started work as a cleaner in the home some time ago and then changed jobs and became a carer. She had been an excellent cleaner and she could have been an excellent carer had she been shown the right way; as it was she worked on a unit where abuse was the normal practice.
There was no real malice in Jackie. I always thought the abuse she committed was the result of ignorance and there was no intent involved in the harm and distress she caused to others.

Jackie would shout at residents in a moment of frustration but her temper would instantly subside. I once came down the corridor and saw Jackie trying to push Margot into unit three dining room. Margot had both hands outstretched and was gripping the door frame so hard it was obvious she had no intention of going through that door for any body. I ran down the hall and asked Jackie why she was doing that. "I am trying to get her to eat and she never wants to come with me" she said indignantly. I asked her to let Margot go as she was in a real state and very distressed, "Just let her walk a lap or two to calm down and then I will show you how to take her in to have her meals." So Jackie let her go and I told Jackie what to do the next time.

Margot passed by again a while later and this time when Jackie saw Margot coming down the hall she stepped out and said to her "Would you like some tea?" and held out the cup in one hand and offered her other arm for Margot to take which she did with a smile and followed Jackie into the dining room and sat and had her meal with no trouble at all.
At first Jackie was amazed at what happened and then she was pleased at how she had done this.

Another time I asked Jackie why she had not given a resident their prescribed laxative and she replied that they would make a mess and she would then have to clean it up. I asked Jackie if she had ever suffered constipation herself and she forgot herself, as some people tend to do when asked about their health, and she launched into a detailed account of a holiday she had once taken abroad and how she had been in absolute agony with constipation and how the pain was so bad her friends had thought she was dying and had called a doctor. I let her continue with the story and when she finally finished I asked her "Why do you think that resident will not suffer similar agony then?"

Her eyes widened in shock and she said "Oh my God, I never thought about it like that." That pretty much summed Jackie up; she never thought about it at all. But if she had been motivated and guided in the right direction she would have been a very different carer to the one she became, she was the only abuser out of them all that could have been trained.

Nadeen was one of little Maria's inner circle of abusers. She was a small blond woman in her forties who had started work at Isard House shortly after Little Maria became team leader. Though Nadeen and Maria both deliberately abused residents they each abused for totally different reasons. Maria abused because she needed to feel the power that came from inflicting pain and fear. Nadeen however did not endow her victims with the capacity to feel at all. To her they were not even human and were only part of the many tasks that had to be done.

I remember the first time that I ever worked with Nadeen, I asked her to help me walk a resident called Annie to the dining room. Annie needed a person on each side and constant encouragement to walk as her co-ordination was very bad and she simply forgot how to move her feet to walk. And she would stop and look at the staff for guidance. It would have been much quicker to just put her in a wheelchair and wheel her to the dining room, but these short walks several times a day kept Annie mobile and whilst she was mobile she was not at risk of pressure sores and all the other complications that are caused by immobility; so compared with all the benefit's for Annie it was well worth a bit more time and effort to walk with her instead.

Nadeen came with me to get Annie who was asleep in the lounge. I gently stroked her face until she woke and she opened her eyes and said "Ooh hello luvie" and I asked her if she wanted to come for a walk. "Ooh yes luvie" she said already leaning forward in the chair. I was talking Annie through how she was going to stand up now when Nadeen suddenly started talking about her boyfriend. I ignored her and carried on talking to Annie who was now standing and we set off down the hall. Annie would take six or seven steps in quick succession and then suddenly stop and look at the staff, "You are walking Annie, you were going to put your right leg out next remember" I said, and Annie replied "Oh yes that's right I was luvie" and off she would go again. Nadeen ignored Annie and continued to talk which distracted Annie and she tried to go forward without moving her feet a couple of times and nearly fell over, so you really had to concentrate on what you were doing. Once Annie was safely seated in the dining room I explained politely to Nadeen that I did not think it was right to talk over residents' heads. It was not only rude but it nearly caused Annie to fall and we were there for her first. I will never forget the look on Nadeen's face "What does it matter? If she needs that much attention put her in a wheelchair", she said aghast.

At best the residents were either invisible to her or barely tolerated, at worst they were noticed by her if she considered them to be a nuisance. The residents that Nadeen noticed were the ones that she had to punish for causing her inconvenience, so the residents that were invisible were really the lucky ones.

Reg was a new resident on unit three. Nadeen considered him a nuisance and Little Maria considered him easy prey. Reg wore a Catheter bag which had to be emptied at regular intervals by staff as he was unable to do this for himself. If the Catheter bag was not emptied then the urine that filled it would flow back up the tube and put Reg at high risk of infection. Also when the bag was full it dragged on Reg and caused him great pain.

I was always finding Reg in the corridors between units two and three, he would be crying in pain from the Catheter bag that had not been emptied. I would take him and empty the bag. This only took a couple of minutes to do and was no trouble. I would then go and find the staff on unit three. I got used to finding all the staff sitting with Little Maria in the back lounge, watching T.V with the door closed so as not to be disturbed by the distressed and neglected residents who walked the corridors looking for staff to help them. Grace and Reg were always with the residents able to get up and go look for help; poor Grace, her face would light up when she saw me. I would go to the staff and tell them there were residents who needed them. Little Maria rarely spoke but would turn her icy gaze on me before turning away again. One night Nadeen turned around when I told her that I had just emptied Reg's Catheter bag again." I will see to him after Coronation Street, he's a bloody nuisance anyway", she said in response.

I reported this to Carole Jones all the time and I felt disappointed each time she said she needed a bit more evidence before she could act. Meanwhile poor gentle Reg was left in pain hour after hour each day. Nadeen was an experienced carer and Little Maria a qualified nurse; they both knew as well as I did why it was so important to empty Catheters regularly.

Reg died a slow and painful death a few months later. Old people of course die of infections all the time and no one ever questions it; after all he could have caught the infection in many ways, who's to say it was from the urine flowing back up the tube of his catheter on those hundred or so occasions that caused it?

Reg once told me that he had been in the last war and saw many of his comrades killed. He said that had he known what he was to face in Isard House, he would not have swam out to a small boat that came to rescue them, it was one of many small boats that came. That made me sad but most of all it made me feel ashamed of my country.

Shouting at residents was second nature to Nadeen. Unlike Jackie who occasionally lost control and shouted in a moment of frustration, Nadeen was always in total control and the residents on the receiving end of her verbal abuse were considered in need of it. How long these tirades went on for was a decision Nadeen made long before she opened her mouth.

Grace, being the one who always tried to help the other residents by fetching the staff, was the one who suffered the most. Every time I heard Nadeen shouting I would run to unit three. I would find Grace flat against a wall flinching from Nadeen whose face would be inches away as she spat a torrent of abuse at her. When I called out Nadeen would turn and Grace, pale and shaking, would escape with a grateful glance at me. Little Maria was never far away and her eyes would narrow and challenge me. I would tell Nadeen I was reporting her and to keep away from Grace. I did go and report it to Carole, each time praying it would be enough to stop it happening any more.

Maria fed off Nadeen's abuse and her enjoyment of it was evident. Nadeen only needed an opportunity and excuse to abuse and little Maria supplied her both in abundance. I dreaded to think what Nadeen was like behind closed doors for that's where most abuse is committed and it's rare to see abuse committed openly in the corridors of a Care Home. I realised as time went on that the complacency was growing as the abusers felt safe to pursue their hobbies.

Jessie was one of Little Maria's prime targets. Maria's control of her was absolute, she moved Jessie into the back lounge and there she was left all day. All the lounges in the home had special high back armchairs for the residents to sit in as these chairs are designed to help residents get up and down from them more easily then a conventional armchair. The back lounge on unit three only contained a few of these special chairs and they were used mainly by the staff as the residents were allocated two sofas. These sofas were used as a very effective form of restraint by Little Maria, who would remove and hide the padded cushions which meant the sofas were then much too low for elderly residents to get up from.

Residents such as Jessie were then left to sit on the hard wooden base from nine in the morning until late that night, up to twelve hours a day every single day. At first they would struggle to get up but after a while you could see the fight go out of them and they would only occasionally raise an arm in silent supplication.

Whenever Jessie's daughter came and asked about the missing cushions, Little Maria would say they were soiled and had been sent to the laundry and that Jessie was safe where she was for a while. Maria was very credible and people did fall for her tactics and that's no reflection on them as Little Maria was just such a good actress. She needed to be or she would not have got away with over twenty years of working in care doing what she did for a hobby.

Little Maria knew her victims well and she also knew when their relatives were likely to visit. I often heard her saying to relatives with a sweetly innocent smile, "Do you work? Oh there must be a lot of hours in that job."

I would often find Jessie in urine saturated clothing, the kind of saturation that takes many hours. Little Maria would put down sheets to protect the base of the sofa, as the sofa was valued more then Jessie's skin. When Jessie saw someone approach she would use the only word she could still utter. "Rose" she would wail in a pitiful cry for help. Little Maria once caught me with Jessie and she spat at me "Get out, she's mine, mine." I had thought Maria was beyond shocking me with her cruelty but looking at her twisted hateful face I knew then that there really was such a thing as evil because I was looking at it.

For the first time in my life I forgot a family birthday. It was my husband Steve's birthday and I was so distracted I completely forgot all about it.

Time passed unbearably slowly and I continued to

report everything to Carole Jones. There was a permanent lump in my throat and I could hardly sleep. I had always got on really well with all the other staff in the home but Carole Jones had made me swear not to talk about the abuse and this was hard but I trusted her and I never confided in anyone. It might have been easier to bear if I had talked to someone else about it.

The corridors on one side of unit two led onto unit three and some of the bedrooms were visible from a certain vantage point. Both units shared the same sluice room which was on unit three.
One early shift I had gone to use this sluice room on unit three when I was struck by this terrible smell. I knew the bins for used pads were kept in the sluice and that it sometimes smelt if it was not emptied but this smell was completely different. I had never smelt anything like this before. Jessie's room was opposite and the door was slightly ajar. As I approached the room Nadeen was suddenly in front of me barring my way. I asked her what the smell was and she said she could not smell anything at all. I caught sight of Jackie who was standing a little way up the corridor, she was shifting from foot to foot in an uncomfortable manner and she could barely bring herself to make eye contact. Nadeen would not move and glanced quickly at Jackie and in that instant I quickly went around her and entered Jessie's bedroom.

As soon as I entered the room I knew it was the

source of the smell. I saw Jessie in the bed and knew that something was really wrong, she was so dehydrated that every vein in her body was clearly visible and grotesquely bulging, her lips were cracked and her tongue so swollen she could barely utter "Rose." The sheets were stained in urine the most recent of which was yellow and soaking wet and the older urine stains dry and stiff, stains in varying shades of yellows and browns which bore witness to how long her torment had lasted this time.

It was not the filth she was left lying in that was the source of the smell I sought. When I turned Jessie gently onto to her side, on the base of her spine there was an open gaping wound so deep the bone was visible; black gangrenous flesh showed where the most recent skin and muscle had rotted and died; an old dressing lay on the sheet near her feet, stained in the pus of infection and too soaked in urine to stick to the skin; around the open wound more signs of skin breaking down, the acid burning already burnt skin and entering the already infected wound. The stench that came from Jessie was a smell that should never issue from the living it; was the smell of decay after death.

They call such open wounds "bed sores." Sore is a sorry description for it goes nowhere near describing the agony of pain that is suffered. I hope to God as long as I live that I never see in another's eyes what I saw in Jessie's.

Beyond The Facade

I ran for Carole Jones and she was a long time with Jessie and then she came and told me she would be alright but that I should not go back in the room as Little Maria would be alerted to the fact that she was about to be sacked. Carole promised me that Jessie would be safe now and that she would be acting very soon, and I believed her, God forgive me.

Sarah Conway was a care assistant on unit three and was one of little Maria's inner circle of abusers. Sarah was in her late twenties, was tall and thin with long brown hair. She had worked in the home sometime, nearly always on the dementia unit's. In all the time I worked in Isard House I had only ever worked a couple of shifts with Sarah but I always felt instinctively uneasy around her.

Aimee was a resident on unit two. She had advanced dementia and was totally dependent on the staff. Everyone loved Aimee, she was gentle and loving and greeted everyone with "Come and have a cuddle." Aimee was just bursting with love and affection, she had been a child minder for many years and also had a large family of her own but Aimee had plenty of love to go round. You could see why she was so loved by all who knew her. She had this maternal warmth about her that drew you to her.

Eileen Chubb

I had just started working on unit two when two of Aimee's daughters came and asked to speak to me. They said all the other staff on the unit knew about their instructions and because I had just started working there I should know also. They seemed so deadly serious that I was beginning to wonder what on earth they were going to say. They then told me that, under no circumstances what so ever, was Sarah Conway ever to be let near their Mother. For a moment I did not know what to think and I said "You do know Sarah Conway has moved to unit three." They said yes they knew, but they still found her on this unit sometimes, and for that reason they wanted me to be aware of the situation. I asked them what had happened and they would only say that I should watch Aimee the next time Sarah Conway came towards her.

A short while after this conversation I was sitting in the lounge on unit two next to Aimee helping her drink her tea as she could no longer hold the cup herself when Sarah Conway entered the room and asked me if I had seen a particular resident from unit three. On catching sight of Sarah, Aimee had flinched back in total fear and then covered her face with her hands and started sobbing violently. I noticed some of the other residents in the room also reacted to Sarah's presence with fear. Sarah looked at Aimee and said "She does that with everyone, she's really confused you know." But I did not believe her because I had seen that degree of fear before; it was there in the eyes of

the residents on unit three every time Little Maria
walked into a room.
Sarah reminded me of Maria in many other ways;
she enjoyed power and it was her motivation to
abuse.

Margot and Ivy had both died. I never got the
chance to say goodbye to Margot but when I
heard Ivy was dying I asked for permission to go
and say goodbye to her. When I arrived on the
unit I found Ivy's bedroom door was open and
from the hallway I could see that Ivy lay quietly in
her bed, her skin already had the smooth sallow
texture that said death was near. She lay still yet
she was alert, her blind eyes following the sounds
and movements in the room. Ivy was not alone.
Little Maria and Sarah Conway were there and
both turned hostile eyes towards me when I
entered. I said that I had permission to see Ivy and
they both turned their eyes towards Ivy as if
noticing her for the first time and they then turned
their backs and continued with their activities.

Ivy's bed was littered with the jewellery and
trinkets that used to be on top of her dressing
table in a large box, her photographs and clothes
were all over the floor. I caught a glimpse of a
photograph I had seen before; it was of a little girl,
her hair a mass of ringlets, wearing a long dress
with an apron over the front. There was a loud
thud as another pile of belongings landed on the
floor scattering everywhere and obscuring the little
girl in the photograph. The wooden rosary beads

that had been in Ivy's bedside cabinet now lay on the floor almost hidden. I picked them up and put them in Ivy's hands, she felt them frantically for a moment and then held them tightly to her chest. I bent down and kissed her forehead and said "God bless Ivy, sweet dreams" and her head nodded almost imperceptibly and then her eyes moved towards the noise as the contents of an old suitcase was tipped out onto the floor. I left the room and went to the office, Ivy died before I got there. She was not even allowed to die in peace, she had no relatives and she left this world whilst two predators took the last thing they could from her.

I found Doris lonely and sobbing, walking the corridors and I took her back to unit two with me. I thought she might get on with Pat, one of the residents I had got to know. I sat Doris next to Pat and asked Pat to look after her for me whilst I made us all a cup of tea. When I returned I found they were both happily chatting away; from then on they spent every single day together and were inseparable. Doris was transformed by this friendship. It was hard to believe the happy animated women sitting talking and laughing with her friend was not so long ago a women that was so desperately lonely she was in constant despair. I asked if Doris could move to unit two and it was agreed.

I would take Doris to her new bedroom to get her washed and dressed for bed. I knew she got up in the night looking for a drink so I always made sure she had one on her bedside cabinet, once she was in bed and comfortable I would wish her a goodnight and she always put her hand up to my face and said "You are my angel you are." If it were not for such moments I could not have gone on. By now the situation on unit three was so bad that I was having the same nightmare over and over again; the residents hands were all I could see and they were all being washed down some kind of underground sewer and I was desperately trying to get hold of their hands and pull them back.

They say like attracts like and there must be some truth in that as Little Maria had attracted every abuser in the home. The staff on my unit was brilliant and I felt lucky in that way. I knew that the residents on unit two were clean, happy and well looked after all the time and that the team on my unit would care for them.

Renee was a senior carer and had worked in the home many years. I had worked with her many times and knew she was a brilliant carer. I had not been working as a team leader on unit two very long when Renee came to work on the unit. She had demoted herself from senior carer on unit three and asked for a transfer. I knew there had been some trouble between Renee and Little Maria, Renee never said what had happened and Carole Jones said that no one should ask about it. Renee settled in well on unit two and all the residents loved her. I felt lucky to have Renee in my team as she was such an excellent carer, one of the best carers in the home, but I worried about the residents on unit three even more now that Renee was not there.

Each unit had their own team leader and a senior carer who acted as deputy. Maggie Roffy was my senior; she had not worked in the home very long when she was promoted. She was an excellent carer and we worked really well together and both had the same approach to the job, in that we were there firstly for the residents and nothing else came before them.

The food that was sent into the home at lunchtime was the only meal the care staff did not have to cook themselves. This food was often no better then slop, grey bits of meat indistinguishable from the pieces of grey vegetables floating in a sea of grey coloured water topped by circles of grease floating on the surface. Maggie and I would see what we could cook from the tins in the store cupboard or failing that we would go halves and one of us would drive to the local shops for food. We could not eat the food that was sent in so there was no way we would feed it to our residents.

We arranged activities for all our residents including an art class. Paper and pens were all donated by relatives and the Christmas of 1998 the residents made every decoration that festooned the unit and they would point out which was their particular masterpiece to all those who visited unit two. Karen was a new carer and was a music and movement instructor so I would offer to make all the beds and clean on my own so that she could do a exercise class with the residents at least twice a week, the sound of their laughter kept me going when I thought I would never finish making all those beds.

We had a beauty and manicure morning and had a big box full of nail varnish, make-up and face packs that the staff and relatives donated, and we would sit in unit two lounge and talk and laugh with the residents as we painted nails and applied make-up, the residents would tell us all about themselves and the funniest stories came out and everyone screamed with laughter, we laughed so much one morning in particular that Carole Jones came down from the office and told us off about the noise.

If ever a unit was alive unit two was, we had this old record player and Maggie got half a dozen L.Ps for 50p each from the charity shop and it's amazing the fun seventeen people can have for under a fiver. One song became a tradition at tea time, all the residents would be sat at the dining tables some already laughing in anticipation and on would go the Mary Poppins L.P and the song "I love to laugh" it was contagious and all the residents roared with laughter while the staff did a maypole dance around an old mop, every time I hear that song I can hear their laughter, God it was just priceless.

Linda Clark was a carer she was bank staff which meant she worked on all the unit's, Linda was another great carer all the residents loved her and she always liked working on my unit, she never said why exactly but I should have known something was wrong when she started bringing the half dead plants from unit three, looking back I can see she was trying to salvage what living thing she could from Maria's grasp.

On unit three little Florie had now been moved into the back lounge to take the place of Jessie, who still lingered between life and death in her bedroom and would not die from the infection for another few months. Flories eyes no longer shone, her spirit seemed to be broken and when someone entered the room her eyes used to look up bright with interest. Now those same eyes looked up in fear.

Some time later I was working an on call shift and had to take the place of one of the night staff who went sick. The report given by the day staff from each unit included the information that Florie was sick and had been for some time with some kind of infection that had taken hold and was not responding to Antibiotics. I waited until little Maria retired to her bedroom upstairs and then went down to check on Florie, I gave her a drink which I noticed she held in her mouth before swallowing. I thought perhaps her mouth might be dry so I went and fetched some Glycerine swabs. It took me well over an hour and dozens of swabs to remove the thick concealed coating of muck, food and dozens of capsules and tablets that lined every inch of her mouth. When I had finished I gave her a drink and she swallowed it and blinked at me she seemed much more comfortable and slept. If Florie had received any treatment for her infection then I doubt it went any further then her mouth, most of the medication I could not identify so had no idea what it was, Florie died the following night.

Since that day, I had gone to Carole Jones and told her about the abuse in front of Little Maria. I did not feel safe. Big Maria the deputy had not spoken to me since that day and it was not long before the staff numbers on my unit were reduced. Where once there had always been nine staff in the home, three staff on each unit, that was now cut back to eight and it was always my unit that was left with only two staff every shift. I went to Carole Jones about this but nothing changed in spite of her assurances. Big Maria had always done the staff rotas and she continued to be in charge of them. Unit three was never short staffed, in fact it was mostly over staffed as Little Maria was not counted in the three staff and that meant there were four staff on duty. Of course if any one said anything Little Maria just said she was not on duty.

I was working a late on call shift and I went to the

office to check if the holiday I had booked was on the rotas as I did not trust Big Maria with it. I found a set of rotas and when I started to flick through them I could see there was something very wrong with them. I looked around and found another set of sheets for the same dates, when I cross checked them I saw nine staff were being paid and yet there were only eight on the rota that really worked. The extra member of staff being paid to make up the staff ratio on my unit was Little Maria. She was being paid for double shifts seven days a week. I spoke to Carole Jones the next day and asked her about this and she said the first set of rotas were only to show the home inspectors and were not real and that only eight staff were being paid. She went into a great big complicated explanation that sounded so confusing that I could not understand what she meant so I left it at that, but the more I thought about it the more sure I was of what I had seen. My suspicions were to be proved well founded.

One morning I was working an early shift and getting the residents up and was on my way to the sluice room when I heard Little Maria shouting "Look at your mess." I stood still almost afraid to look and then I saw Florence C appear with Little Maria just behind her, Maria then drew back her arm as far as it would go and hit Florence hard in the back. The force of the blow caused Florence to fall forward in to her bedroom and out of my view. Before Little Maria followed into the room I caught a glimpse of her face for a second, it reminded me of someone watching something like the Grand National with that same mixture of anticipation and excitement, but there was also something else something that was twisted, as usual I went to Carole.

Lena was a resident on unit two, she was in her early eighties and walked with a Zimmer frame. When I first came to work on the unit I noticed that Lena was asleep a lot of the time and would only get up from her armchair to look for the toilet. I found out that Lena got really distressed when staff tried to take her to her bedroom at night to get her ready for bed and because of this Lena was left to sit in the lounge until the night staff put her to bed in the early hours of the morning and with the same level of distress that the day staff had tried to avoid. I watched Lena closely and noticed that when the staff were putting other residents to bed, Lena would get up around the same time each evening and look for the toilet. When she next got up I was ready and waiting and had prepared her bedroom in advance, bedclothes turned down, curtains closed, the light on and the commode with the lid up ready, I knew Lena needed the toilet and would not go into a dark room so this all helped. When she got up I asked her if she needed the toilet and she said yes and followed me to her bedroom. Once there I said to her that she might as well get washed and put her nightdress on as it was getting late and it would save her a job later. Lena happily agreed, so I got her washed properly and helped her into her nightclothes. I said I would go and get her a milky drink and left her sitting in her armchair, when I came back with a hot drink Lena had gotten into bed, "Was a bit tired" she said. After that Lena went to bed and was washed and cared for every night. She no longer slept during the day and joined in all the activities, in fact it was often Lena who laughed the loudest.

Mary was a resident on unit two. She was quite independent and mobile and only had mild dementia. Mary could wash and dress herself and only needed a bit of guidance, the only thing she could not manage was getting her stockings on, but she only wore them on special occasions. One day Mary came and asked if the staff could help with her stockings on Saturday as she was going out with her family to a wedding. Saturday came and when I came on duty at lunchtime I found only one member of staff on unit two and asked where the other one was. The carer told me that they had been left on their own to get on with it. I could see this carer was exhausted. I couldn't believe that they would leave one girl to do everything and asked who had gone sick and they said no one was sick. The other member of staff that was supposed to be working on unit two had been sent to unit three instead. I went down to unit three and found four staff including Little Maria who was sitting in a armchair reading the newspaper. I asked what was going on and she glared at me and said she was not on duty. There was nothing I could do so I walked back to my unit and with a heavy heart. I saw Mary walk of with her son, she was not wearing her tights and she told me later she did not want to ask the girl on duty as she could see she was run ragged. Poor Mary never asked for anything and the one day she needed help she did not get any because Little Maria wanted to sit and get paid for it. I felt like crying it was bad enough what was happening to the residents on unit three and there was no way I would allow any one else to suffer as well.

I was working a late shift and had gone into the kitchen on unit two and turned on the light. The serving hatch to the dining room was open and through it I could see the outline of someone sitting at a table. The dining room was in darkness apart from the light from the kitchen and the little light that came through the glass partition on the other side of the room, so I was unable to make out who it was sitting there.
I walked around and turned on the lights, it was Dot, she looked relieved to see me and then she quickly looked around and told me to turn the lights off. She seemed really frightened so I turned them off as I did not want to worry her any more. I asked her what she was doing there sitting in the dark and she said "It's them two women they keep hurting me and I don't want them to find me." I was about to ask her more when Little Maria and Nadeen went to pass by in the hallway on the other side of the glass partition, they caught sight of me standing there with the light from the serving hatch behind me and then they both saw Dot and

walked around and entered the room. Dot froze in fear when she saw them "It's them two please don't let them take me", she pleaded with me, my heart was pounding and I desperately tried to keep my voice calm as I turned to Little Maria and said "I can put Dot to bed for you if you like I am ahead with my own work." Nadeen stayed just inside the doorway and Little Maria crossed over to where I was standing and spat at me in almost a whisper "She's mine", she called Nadeen over and they stood either side of Dot and took her with them. Dot looked back at me once just before she left the room her eyes pleading with me. I stood there numb for another minute or so and then felt this overwhelming despair and sadness. I knew I could not get all the residents from unit three on to my unit and then run up and down shouting Sanctuary like some kind of demented Quasi Modo. The fact that such a thought had even occurred to me made me realise I was closer to breaking point then ever before, I mentally reminded myself to trust Carole, it won't be long now.

A little while later I was working a late shift when the emergency bleep I was carrying went off. It was from unit three which was very unusual. I ran down and saw that Dot had fallen in the doorway of the lounge. Little Maria was leaning over her and her eyes narrowed when she saw me. "She is not injured go back to your own unit "she said through clenched teeth. I told her I would just help her lift Dot and then I will go, then Dot grabbed me with both hands and cried, "Please don't leave me with her, please." Dot was pleading with me as if her life depended on it and hanging on to my arm tighter then ever. Little Maria then started screaming "Get off my unit now or you will be in big trouble." I had no choice but to leave, I had to take Dot's hands off my arm while she pleaded with me not to leave her with Maria. I will never forget the fear in her eyes and I will never forgive myself for walking away from a friend who needed my help.

The next morning as soon as Carole Jones came through the door I went to her but Little Maria had got to her first as her friend Big Maria had phoned Carole the night before. Carole said I was not to go on to unit three and she watched me intensely as if trying to read my expression. "You do trust me don't you? It will soon be over", she said.

I was working a late shift and Amanda the team leader from unit one was in charge of the home that night. I was in the lounge on unit two when Amanda came and asked me to do the medication on unit three. Little Maria had taken one of her very rare nights off so there was no one else to do it. I could not tell Amanda that I was supposed to stay off the unit as she would want to know why, so reluctantly I went. When I reached unit three lounge Jackie was already waiting with the medication trolley. It was the normal practice for the senior member of staff to dispense the dose of medication and watch while a junior member of staff administered it to the resident and once the medication was swallowed I would sign that it was given. I gave two residents their medication and turned to the next sheet which was Edna's, her sheet stated 10mls of Chlorpromazine three times daily, so I measured out the evening dose of 10mls and passed it to Jackie, who looked at it and said immediately, "That's not right. Maria always gives her a lot more then that." I double checked the G.P instructions again and 10mls three times a day was clearly stated then I looked to the other of side and saw that that doses of 30mls three time a day had been given for weeks, these doses of 90mls a day were signed for by Little Maria. Chlorpromazine is a very powerful Anti-psychotic drug and has to be used with even more caution when the patient is elderly. This is because elderly people can often have impaired renal function and drugs can not easily be flushed out of the system so they are at a higher risk from drugs building up in their system to lethal levels. That is why the drug Chlorpromazine's recommended upper safe limit for an elderly patient is set at 40mls a day.

"Where's Edna?" I said to Jackie who pointed to the corner table, I got up and went over, Jackie followed me looking really worried as she had picked up on the panic in my voice. Jackie became more agitated by the minute and said," I am never doing the drugs with Maria again she never gives them the right ones it's not me. I only do what she says."

I looked at Edna who was sleeping with her head

on the table, I told Jackie I was going for the on-call officer and Jackie became distraught and started wringing her hands and continued to disown any blame. "Maria tells me what to give. It's not me. She gave a residents Dioxin to someone else you know." Dioxin is a drug given to slow the heart it can potentially stop the heart if overdosed. Amanda ran back with me and I explained all as we went. She ran to check Edna and we got her to her bedroom and Amanda got someone to stay with her. She looked at the medication sheets and at the bottles in the trolley and then wrote out a detailed report of the whole thing on sheets of paper and got me to sign it with her as a witness. She put it in a sealed envelope addressed to Carole Jones. "I can not write it in the report book or Big Maria will see it", she said and went back to Edna.

Kitty was a resident on unit three, she came to live in the home after I had left unit three the first time so I did not know her as well as the other residents, but I really liked her as she was always so cheerful in spite of having curvature of the spine and severe arthritis. That meant she had such a high level of pain that the doctor prescribed her really strong pain relief to be given every four hours so that the pain could be kept at a level she could bear. Little Maria saw the potential of this and she withheld the pain relief from Kitty and watched her suffer. Maria did not even order this medication and falsified the medication sheets to conceal the prescription existed just in case another member of staff gave it to her by mistake. It did not take long before Kitty's screams could be heard so Little Maria took her into the back lounge and closed the door. One evening Little Maria had gone out and was not expected back until later. I was the on-call officer that evening and Lee came round from unit three and asked me to come and look at Dot. "She is still very sick", he said. This was the first time I was made aware of it and told Lee that there was nothing in the handover book about Dot being sick. I went with Lee and he explained as we walked around to Dot's room that he had asked Little Maria to call a doctor and that she had promised she would but no doctor has come he said. I remembered Iris and I wondered if Lee had waited for Maria to leave in case she saw him speaking to me, but I dared not ask him as Carol had been adamant I should speak to no one about Maria and I did not know Lee well enough to risk it. When we arrived at Dot's room I found her in bed sitting up, she was really pale and clammy and was gripping her stomach in terrible pain. I knew she was in a bad way and immediately rang the emergency doctor. While I waited for the doctor to arrive I checked Dot's records, there was a request for a doctor to visit made some weeks earlier but Little Maria had written "Not Needed" over the top and cancelled it and after that there was no mention of any pain or sickness. I knew Dot had a history of severe constipation so I checked her medication sheets next. Half of her medication was not even entered on the sheets so it had not been ordered and it had not been stopped by the G.P. The remaining medication was in the trolley but had never even been opened or administered. The doctor came and examined Dot and prescribed the medication that she should have been given all along, he said that she was so badly constipated it blocked her whole bowel and that the district nurses would have to come in daily to administer enemas. I went to Carole as usual and she said she would carry out a full drugs audit and that I needed to be patient a little longer as it would take a little more time to complete. I never doubted for a second that Carole would find all the evidence she needed to sack Little Maria.

Abbey was a resident on unit three, Little Maria told everyone she had gone on holiday with her daughter. I went to speak to Carole Jones one afternoon and found her in the conference room writing in a residents care plan. I saw that it was Abbey's care plan and I must have looked puzzled as Carole started to explain what she was doing and said that Abbey's daughter had removed her from the home and that she was going to sue Carole for the abuse her Mother had suffered in the home. "We have to stick together it's me she will sue and who will get rid of Maria if I am gone?" she said by way of an explanation. I could see that Carole was re-writing sections of the care plans and that amounted to falsifying them. I felt really uneasy for the first time but I was so desperate to believe she would stop the abuse that I could not comprehend her doing otherwise.

Eileen Chubb

My residents and staff on unit two had suffered badly because I had risked reporting the abuse to Carole Jones. My staffing levels were cut to the bone. We worked flat out and were lucky to even get a break and even then we could not leave the unit and go to the staff room as it would only leave one member of staff alone on the unit with seventeen residents, many of whom needed two members of staff to lift them. So we made the best of a bad situation and had our breaks on a bench outside the fire exit which meant we could be called if needed and as this bench was right next to the lounge window so we could also keep an eye on the residents. It was really cold in the winter sitting out there but it was better than no break at all so we kept a fleece top hanging in the kitchen which was shared by all the staff.

I was sitting on that bench one lunchtime when Lee came out and asked if he could speak to me, he kept looking around nervously checking no one else could hear then he said, he was seeing the most terrible abuse on unit three and that it was getting worse and he could bear it no longer. He spoke very quickly that it was as if he had held it in so long that he could not speak fast enough. I had to tell him to slow down at one point because he was hardly drawing breath. He took a couple of deep breaths and continued but it was not long before I stopped him again as what he was telling me was so serious I said he must go to Carole right now and tell her this. I trusted her even then and still thought she would act especially now another witness was willing to come forward. When Lee said he had already gone to Carol and had been going to her for ages I thought I had misheard him at first and then everything slowed down. I felt like I had been punched hard and it took my breath away, I was there looking at Lee and could see his mouth moving and yet it was all in slow motion, distorted like in a bad dream. It was like I was watching from afar and then I suddenly snapped back into focus as Lee told me how Carole had said she needed him to collect more evidence to sack to Maria and how Maria could get a job somewhere else. She also said she would abuse again, how he should help her collect evidence to sack Maria and that he should not speak about it to anyone else. Lee said how he had gone to Carole again and again and that he had been told to trust her, so had the others. "Others there are others?" I shouted and he said Renee and Linda and young Lizzy had all gone too and that he had just found out about them and that was why he was coming to me. "What are we going to do?" he asked me. I told him I needed to speak to the others and that I would do something about it, but Renee was off and I told him to wait until she came back. I promised Lee I would do something but I did not know what and I needed to think.

I spent the rest of that day going over everything that had happened, all the times I had gone to Carole, I could see her face clearly as she told me to trust her. I remembered all the times I had gone to her but most of all I remembered the suffering I had reported and I felt numb at first and as the reality of it sunk in I felt sick. When Renee came back to work I spoke to her and she told me everything, how she could bear the abuse no longer and had asked Carole to demote her and transfer her off unit three. She said she had been sworn to secrecy by Carole who promised she would act "I trusted her like a bloody fool" she said.

The next day I was on a late shift and I walked on to unit two in time to help serve lunch and do the medication. Maggie was there and she said that Little Maria had done the morning medication and had not given two of the residents their drugs but had signed them as given on the sheet.

Maggie was worried about how to return the drugs and rightly so, as the medication on unit two was well managed, so well managed we did not even need to use the cupboard in the medication room that was allocated for storage. Each unit had a cupboard and drug trolley but as a new team leader on unit one, I had discovered that drugs left in the cupboard went missing. It did not take long to discover where these drugs had gone. Little Maria had access to these cupboards but not the drugs trolleys, so I spent more time on my orders and got it exactly right so everything could be kept in the trolley. I trained Maggie to keep the medication in good order and she knew only the right way of doing things. If drugs were not administered they were supposed to be returned by entering in a small box a letter code for the reason they were not given. There was a small box for each date where you signed that you had given the drugs or you returned them by entering a code letter which explained why the drugs had not been given, in short there was only room for a signature or a return as it would be impossible to return what you had administered. I told Maggie I would go and ask Carole how to return these drugs, Carole was off for a couple of days but the drugs did not need to be returned to the chemists until Friday and Carole would be back at work before then. As soon as Carole returned I went to the office and asked to speak to her, she said she was busy and that I should come back after lunch, which I did and we went to the conference room. It was 2pm on April 15th 1999. I had taken the medication sheets with me so I showed them to Carole and asked how to return the medication, she told me to write the code R which meant the medication had been refused by the resident. I said that would mean I would have to write over Little Maria's signature which would conceal it and it would be falsifying the medical records. Carole repeated that I was to do that anyway. I looked at her in silence for a couple of minutes, I knew she was an accessory in the abuse by now but I just needed to hear the words come from her own mouth, the same mouth that had promised to stop the abuse so many times. I felt unnaturally calm and when I spoke it did not even sound like my voice. I told Carole that I would take no part in forging medical records and then I asked what she had found on the drug audit she had carried out. She said there was nothing wrong at all and no more would be said about it. I knew the medication records on unit three showed clear evidence of abuse, so clear no one with half a brain could fail to see it. There was no way that a qualified nurse like Carole could fail to see what was going on. I stood up slowly and said "I now understand" and I walked away. I could hear Carole saying "Eileen come back we can be reasonable about this." God I thought she thinks I would negotiate on it like it was some kind of disagreement over how to make the beds or something. I went back to my unit and finished what little time was left of my shift and when Maggie asked about the drugs being returned I said "Carole said we should write R for refused in the return box" Maggie looked horrified and said it would be forgery and I told her it was alright we would not be doing it and that we would talk tomorrow. I went home in a daze I already knew what I had to do there was no choice involved. I told Steve my husband about everything for the first time, I had not dared tell him before as I knew he would make me leave but he said he knew something was wrong, I had been distracted all the time and he had thought I was tired at first. We were most definitely not in a financial position for me to risk losing my job, but Steve immediately said he would support me every step of the way and that I had to report it what ever happened. He was true to his word and has supported me all the way, then at the very start and through all the hardship that was to follow.

The next day was Friday April 16th 1999 and I was due to work an early shift before my four days off. I went to work and during the course of that morning I spoke to Maggie, Linda, Lee, Lizzy, Karen and Renee and I told them each in turn that I was going to Bromley Social Services on Monday morning. I said if they wanted to write a statement about the abuse they had seen that I would take it with me, but as they would be risking their jobs in doing so I told them that I would not blame them if they chose to say nothing. Each of those six carers said immediately they would write a statement for me to take. Not one of them hesitated for a second, I felt so privileged to work with these people, people who cared enough to risk everything to speak out. If I had a care home then I would be proud to employ such people. Looking back we would all have made exactly the same choices again, even had we known what was to follow, for we were about to bring the might of a multi-national Company down upon us with such fury that to this day we still ask why?

That weekend was spent writing out my statement it was the biggest thing I had written since leaving school, the only writing I had done since was an occasional letter to the bank about direct debit's or similar. I started to panic that I would never get it written down by Monday. There was so much to cram into it that it would fill a book and I only had two days to write it all. Steve could see how worried I was getting and said just write down a summary of what's happened for now and you can always tell them the rest verbally. When I read that statement now I can see how much emotion and turmoil I felt. It's there in the blotches of ink smudged by the tears that came when I remembered what I had seen. Very little of the person who wrote that statement remains for I was about to begin a fight that would turn my world upside down for ever. I had arranged to meet with the other six carers early on Monday morning to collect their statements. We met at the end of the road that led to Isard House, when I arrived they were all waiting. It was still cold at that time of the morning and Lizzy stood shivering, her teeth chattering as she stamped her feet trying to keep warm. Everyone had their statements ready and handed them to me, I said I would go and photo copy them in case we had to go to the press, by this point we hoped that Social Services would stop the abuse but we had waited for so long for that to happen that we trusted no one and had discussed going to the press as a secondary plan if Social Services failed to help us. Karen worked the same shift pattern as me so she was also off work and said she would come with me. The others waited in Renee's car until their early shift started except Lizzy who was due to work a late shift so went back home to wait, It was five thirty on the morning of Monday April 19th 1999. I went to a nearby newsagent and made copies of all the statements and then went to wait at Karen's house. I tried to eat some toast but could not swallow more then a mouthful and paced up and down looking at the clock waiting for the time to pass. Karen lived within walking distance of Bromley Civic Centre where Social Services were based so she knew how long it would take to walk there. Finally it was time to set of which was a relief as the waiting was the worst part. We arrived at Bromley Civic Centre just as the doors opened. I took all of the statements out of my bag and held them ready, took a deep breath and walked in. I saw a reception desk and went over, I noticed the two receptionists carried on talking to each other and ignored me standing there and dozens of receptionists had done that to me in the past and I normally would have just stood there and waited patiently. "Excuse me, while I am standing here waiting for you to notice me elderly people are most likely being abused and whatever you are talking about it can not be as important as that. So can you get someone from Social Services so I can hand over these statements about abuse and torture and can you do that right now", I heard a loud determined voice say and then I realised it was me that had spoken and I thought God whatever came over me making a scene like that and I felt my cheeks burning. Within a couple of minutes a lady came out of the lift and hurried over, she said her name was Monica Handscomb and that she was a home inspector. She took us over to a small side room and has soon as we sat down she said," What Home is it?" I told her it was Isard House and that we were two of the care staff and had brought statements from five other staff also. I went to pass her the thick pile of statements and she took hold of them but I found I could not let go of them as I said, "I have copies of these and I will take them to the press if the abuse is covered up" as we both gripped the statements. Karen like a delayed echo said "She has copies and we will go to the press if it's covered up." Monica looked really shocked and said "I promise you no abuse will be covered up. Whatever made you think you could not trust us?" I explained we trusted no one and with a huge effort I managed to bring myself to let go of the statements so suddenly Monica fell back in her chair, finally with the statements in her hands she started to read the first page on the top of the pile but after only a couple of minutes she said" This is really serious I need to get my boss down here" and she used the phone. A couple of minutes later a man entered the room, he was in his late forties and slim built. He introduced himself as Dick Turner and said he was in charge of the Social Services inspection team. He sat down next to Monica listened as she read out a little of the first page, Mr Turner said he and Monica needed some time to read through all the statements and asked if we minded going for a cup of tea which we agreed to and he took us to a large cafeteria and said he would come back for us. We sat there nervously sipping a cup of tea, grateful for a bit of space to talk through what had happened so far. I kept watching the doorway waiting for Mr Turner to come back for us. After some time Mr Turner came and took us back to the same small room, he said "The contents of these statements are of grave concern and the allegations relate to the most serious abuse. An immediate investigation will commence and as the allegations relate to serious criminal offences I will be informing the police "he then went on to say that Monica had told him how she thought it dreadful we felt unable to trust anyone and he assured us there would be no cover-up. He also went on to say it would take a couple days to put together an investigation team and brief them and then they would go to Isard house and fully investigate everything and said as whistle-blowers our identities would be protected and no one would ever have to know who had made the allegations. They both seemed to be very genuine so we agreed to leave it with them for now and said we would wait to hear from them. As soon as we were alone outside I said to Karen "What's a whistle-blower?" "I don't know" she replied "I wonder what the new manager will be like" and I said all that matters is that it's over now the abuse will stop. But it was only the beginning I never imagined that doing the right thing would be so hard. If I had known I would still have done the same thing, I was about to find out the hard way that you do not need a whistle to report abuse you needed a brass band, an army of body guards and a very large bank balance.

I went home and told Steve what had happened and during that day I spoke to the others when they telephoned and told them what had happened. They all asked if we could trust Social Services to act and I told them that I did not know yet but we would have to wait and see what happens in the next two days. I said that we could still go to the press later if nothing was done about the abuse, so we waited.

On the morning of Wednesday 21st of April 1999, Social Services and the police entered Isard House, I was not on duty until that afternoon so did not see Maria Keenahan being arrested and taken out of the home. Sarah Conway was also arrested a short while later. The investigation team took over an old disused flat on the top floor of Isard House it was to be the base for their investigation and where they would interview all the staff. Later on that same day I returned to work after my four days off to work an on-call shift. It was 2pm and I took my overnight bag to the on-call room and went to the office for the report book. As I entered I saw that there were four people in the room, Carole Jones, Big Maria, Linda the secretary and Carole Newton, who I had only seen once or twice before and who was the BUPA Regional Manager. They all looked up as I entered and I said as casually as I could that I needed the report book, they did not speak. So I saw the book on the desk and picked it up and walked out of the room feeling very uncomfortable. I was just through the doorway when I clearly heard Carole Jones say "I told you she would be trouble the amount of times she has come to me" and I thought so much for our identities being kept confidential. I walked quickly down to unit two, I felt better when I got there, and in the weeks that were to follow I learnt there were thirty two steps from the front door to the first section of unit two, just thirty two steps through a wall of hate that became a walk of fear. When I reached the kitchen on unit two Maggie was there and she told me what had happened that morning, and then I felt huge relief at the thought that the residents on unit three would not be abused any more, it's really over. When the late shift finished that night I went to the on-call room where I would spend the night. I did not feel safe anymore and before I lay down I pushed the dressing table in front of the door, then I counted the hours until I could go home.

The night passed slowly and eventually after working an early shift next day I wrote a report of events on my unit in the report book and waited for the staff from the other two units to come and give me their reports. That was the usual procedure that was followed only the staff never came so I had to go to them. I found Dee, a carer on unit one and asked for her handover." I would not hand over any information to you, you would tell that lot upstairs" she spat at me. I walked back to my unit and I felt like crying. I had known Dee a long time and had always got on well with her and would never have imagined that she would behave that way towards me. As I passed other staff in the hallways similar comments were made and that's how it began. The dirty laundry was no

longer collected from our unit, nor was any clean
clothes delivered for our residents, we would have
to walk through a wall of hate to get the laundry
ourselves. We took it in turns and the one whose
turn it was to go would be given looks of pity. I
remember the first time I walked to the laundry,
the staff from the other unit's were suddenly there.
There was a terrible silence at first and then one
or two threats quickly followed by a torrent of
abuse. People I had worked with for years and
who I thought I knew turned into total strangers
that I no longer recognised at all, they became
part of a violent mob whose rage and hate knew
no limit's and they lined the route of those thirty
two steps, shouting, "We are going to lose our
jobs because of you and your tale telling"
"You are going to pay for this you won't get out of
here in one piece" "Wait till it's dark we will get you
in the car park" and "Here come the scum" were
all typical jeers we suffered and behind the mob
the sneering face of Carole Jones and Carole
Newton always beside her making sure we knew
whose side she was on.

They say that sticks and stones can break your
bones but names can never hurt you, it's not true
because I know how it feels to be on the receiving
end of really bad verbal abuse and it hurts you.
The threat of violence and the sheer hatred is hard
to imagine unless you have been in such a
position. It crushes you a little more each day and
when you escape at the end of that day it still
reaches you, for the only thing worse then walking

through the hate to go home, is the fear of what's yet to come when you walk back in the next day, that fear is there all the time, first you do not sleep and then you do not eat until in the end you can not function any more. Every member of staff in the home was interviewed by Social Services over the following weeks. You would be summoned to the flat one at a time and before you climbed the stairs they would see one of the mob standing duty, watching who went in and who came out but most of all how long they were in there. The sentry would make a big show of looking at their watch and everyone knew they were being timed and that the information would be taken back to the office where members of the mob always seemed to be when they should have been caring for their residents.

Carole Newton walked onto unit two several times a day, she stood watching silently and writing notes in a small black book, and then she would walk off smiling and we all knew notes were being made about us and evidence being fabricated because as far as she and BUPA were concerned we were the ones who were the problem. Little Mollie was one of the residents on unit two, one late shift Karen and I had just served the residents tea, when Mollie got up from the table and fell, I rang the emergency alarm as was normal in such a situation and Linda Clark came from unit three and Anne Davidson from unit one. I was on the floor kneeling over Mollie checking her for any injuries when they arrived. Anne Davidson immediately started shouting abuse, Linda and I said nothing for a while and then once I had checked Mollie was unhurt I asked Anne Davidson to bring a chair while Linda helped me lift Mollie up, the next thing I knew I was hit hard in the back, so hard my whole body went forward with the force of the blow and my head went down on Mollies chest. It was not the pain of the blow that got me right then, nor was it Anne Davidson who stood holding the chair she had smashed into my back and who was still screaming abuse "You fucking make me sick you lot", it was not even the sound of the other residents in the room crying. What got me was little Mollie who put her hand up to my face and said "Are you alright duckie?" I started crying then because there was this old women who had fallen on the floor and who was asking me if I was alright. I got up from the floor after a while. There was a large part of me that just wanted to sit there and surrender, I felt like I had no more strength left and than some kind of automatic pilot took over and I got up and carried on, I had no choice my residents needed me. I felt empty as I did what needed to be done. I asked Karen to take the residents several of whom were distraught and crying into the lounge, I went through the rest of the shift in a daze.

When I got home that night Steve took one look at my face and asked me what had happened, it was only then that the full impact of what had happened slammed into me, when I told him about the chair being smashed into my back he stared at me for a minute as if he had not heard me and then he insisted on checking where I had been hit. I have never seen him so angry he went mad when he saw the state of my back, the chair had left a huge welt across my back and the bruising was already coming out. He said "You are not going back in there" and that's when I started to cry because I knew he was right, and than I said, they would win and that's what they wanted to do drive us out so he relented, I wrote out a full account of the assault and gave it to Mr Turner the next day so he could pass it to the Police.

A senior BUPA Director, Des Kelly came and spoke to the staff on unit one and unit three, young Lizzie was on unit three and she overheard him telling staff they had his full support in this difficult time, but he never spoke to Lizzie or any of the staff on unit two who had reported the abuse. He bypassed unit two and made it obvious we did not have the company's support. When I got home I told Steve about it, "What kind of people are you working for?" he said. Linda's husband wanted her to come out of work too, she had been trying to feed Aimee when both the cleaners came into the room and started screaming abuse, then they repeatedly rammed the Hoover into her legs. Dot was in hospital the pain had become too much, I was so upset about Dot. I said when I was interviewed by Social Services that it was Carole Jones fault she was in hospital as she had ignored the abuse. I was devastated when I found out some time later that

Eileen Chubb

Dot had died.

Carole Newton came after me the day of Dot's funeral, I had gone to the funeral in the morning and then gone to work my late shift, Carole Newton was waiting and she said" Carole Jones and I want to talk to you now in the conference room." I told her there was only myself and Maggie on the unit and it was not safe to leave the unit so understaffed, but instead of finding staff to cover me she started following me around trying to physically block me from doing my job. I said "Please I can not do my job like this" and she sneered "Well if you can't do your job we will have to do something about it." I tried to get past her but she kept blocking my path, at one point she nearly knocked a resident over who trying to get past her, but she was oblivious to the residents. I knew it was impossible to work like this so I borrowed Maggie's mobile phone and locked myself into one of the bedrooms. I could hear Carole Newton outside but she went off when she could not get in. I was afraid she had gone to get the spare keys to open the door, I rang Social Services and told them what was happening and that I was locked in a room and needed them to come quickly. Dick Turner and Monica Handscomb did come and later that same day I met with Carole Newton in the conference room with Mr Turner and Monica present. I told her what was happening to us but she seemed hostile throughout, nothing was done to help us, it just got much worse. Lee and Lizzie the two youngest carers were the most vulnerable and were the first to crack under the pressure, they could not go on and went to their G.Ps and were both signed off sick with stress, Lee tried to return to work but the harassment was so bad he was signed off sick for a second time.

It was a late shift and we had seen Carole Jones walking up and down to unit three most of that afternoon, her hands full of medication records she was removing from the unit, we were all worried she was destroying incriminating evidence. I was the on-call officer for the coming night so I would have the keys to the office when Carole Jones and the other office staff left. Maggie went out in her break and bought copier paper and we watched and waited for Carole Jones to go home. Carole walked onto unit two at tea time as I was doing the medication and she threw the heavy bunch of keys at me from the doorway. They missed my head and nearly hit the resident sitting beside me. Carole walked off and I looked at Maggie who was nearby and saw that she was crying so I tried to make light of it and said "That must be the handover then" Maggie smiled but the tears were running down her face and her hands were shaking as she said "Those keys could have hit you or Lena."
After a while we checked the car park to make sure Carole had left for the evening.

I walked to the office and ignored the mob who shouted at me as I passed, it was not unusual for the on-call officer to go to the office for a while so I knew I would have to be quick and then I would not arouse any suspicion.

I went into the office and gathered together all the unit three records that I could find, I put them in a folder and walked out and locked the door and walked back to unit two, as I rounded the corner Renee was waiting, she was working on unit three that night and had timed her break just right. I passed the folder to Renee, who already had the copier paper and she went across the unit and down a back corridor that led to the back stairs which were rarely used and which allowed Renee to get to the photo copier in the upstairs conference room unobserved. She copied all the records and came back down by the same route and I returned the records to the office and we hid the copy's in unit twos bathroom under the towels. We then did the same with the records from the medical room, it was difficult because we were watched so much but we got them out of the room in a medication trolley and even though two of the mob had seen us and started screaming abuse, we didn't think they suspected anything but they must have thought something was wrong because they rang Carole Jones. We had just finished the photo coping and were returning the records to the medical room when Carole Jones was seen pulling into the car park. We ran back to unit two and hid the copies with the others in the bathroom and had reached the kitchen when Carole Jones marched around the corner and demanded that I gave her the keys before marching off, from the other corner Renee watched her and saw her unlocking the door to the medical room. Renee ran to me and said "She's going into the medical room. Oh my God those records will still be hot from the copier."

Those records did turn out to be hot but not in the way Renee meant. If we had not smuggled those records out of the home they would most certainly have been destroyed but we never imagined that the actions we took that night were to prove that a cover-up had taken place, we could not have foreseen how far that cover-up would extend. No doubt Carole Jones did manage to destroy some of the records. In the past Maria Keenahan was seen burning records and that was before the investigation, but the records that we saved were enough to prove beyond any shadow of a doubt, that we were telling the truth and that our employers, BUPA knew that from the start. All the medication records showed the same patterns but it was Edna's records that were to become the most well known.

Grace was left sitting in the lounge all night. Nadeen was afraid it might be noticed how neglected she looked as the inspectors were upstairs during the day. Nadeen took action. She got Jackie to help her carry Grace into her room. Grace was screaming and struggling and all her clothes were torn. She was washed by force and put to bed sobbing. I did see Grace one last time, she was sitting in her room, all her torn clothes laid out on the bed, "I was going to give them to someone who needed them but now there all ruined", she said. I only had time to give her a hug before some of the mob came screaming into the room and I was told to get off that unit. The last thing I heard was Grace sobbing, I never saw her again. She died a few month's later.

The Harassment continued, as time went on it became apparent that the mob consisted of all staff in the home with the exception of only four people, the cleaners and laundry staff were also part of this mob. The management had the power to change your shifts without warning and did so, you would show up to work your usual shift only to be told you were not on the rota, or you would be rung at home and asked why you were not in work when you were not even supposed to be there. Whenever we managed to get a break we would go outside and sit on the bench but we would be jeered at by the mob from the opposite windows. To start with the mob only jeered us as we walked to and from our unit but then it got much worse and they started to come on to unit two, walking up and down screaming abuse and banging the bedroom doors so hard that it frightened our residents. I thought the residents on our unit were also being blamed and were seen as one of "Them" which is how they referred to us.

I met with Carole Newton again and this time someone from BUPA's H.R Department. I told them again about the harassment and still nothing was done. It was if the mob had official approval to do what they were doing but because it was getting worse by the day we all knew we could not go on much longer. I was working an early shift and went in to see Mary, she seemed a bit unwell so I washed her and made her comfortable. When I returned to collect her breakfast tray she had eaten nothing and she became gradually more unwell as the morning went on. I was worried and went to call the G.P and was talking to him on the phone and saw Mary's daughter in law had arrived and overheard me. She said she was glad I had called the doctor as she thought Mary was not quite herself.

I continued with my work and a short while later the unit telephone rang, it was Carole Jones and she said in a very hostile tone, "Why have you called a doctor in?" I said Mary was ill and she needed the doctor, Carole Jones then said, "Why can it not wait until the G.P comes on Friday." I said that it could not wait until the end of the week, then the phone was banged down. The late shift staff overheard the conversation and I told them the G.P would be in today for Mary and to keep a close eye on her, my shift was over and I went home. When I returned the next day to work a late shift and was told by the staff that Mary had collapsed and that a doctor had come and rang an ambulance, I asked what the first doctor had said yesterday and I was told no doctor had come the day before and they had requested the doctor again that morning. After Carole Jones had telephoned me the day before she had cancelled my request for the doctor. Mary had collapsed from an infection that had gone into her kidneys, the G.P who called the ambulance asked why the doctor requested the day before had been cancelled as Mary was so ill and could have been treated a crucial twenty four hours earlier. The staff said he needed to ask Carole Jones as she made that decision. Mary died the next day. She paid the ultimate price for Carole Jones anger at me.

Mary's relatives came in to clear her room a few days later and they thanked me for calling the doctor for Mary so quickly, Carole Jones and Big Maria hovered near the door. Carole's face was covered by a film of sweat and her eyes darted around nervously and she could barely make eye contact, I looked at her long and hard and hoped she knew the absolute disgust I felt, disgust that she could even stand there after what she had done and let Mary's family thank her for the care she received.

Edna, poor gentle Edna, during the subsequent legal proceedings Edna's medication records proved Carole Jones allowed the illegal over-dosing to continue long after she was aware of it and right up to the day Little Maria was arrested. Little Maria enjoyed playing God just as Dr Harold Shipman enjoyed having the power to give life or take it under his control. Little Maria was motivated in exactly the same way and she enjoyed a game of Russian roulette and her preferred weapon of choice was the drug

Chlorpromazine when it came to Edna's life, doses of up 180mls were administered. The last time that I saw Edna she could not walk or talk, I remembered how she loved to have a bath as I smelt the rancid sour smell that I had come to know so well. The stench of deliberate wilful abuse.

Her body jerked constantly from the drug induced Parkinson's that is a side effect of the drug Chlorpromazine and which is irreversible. This same drug in liquid form can burn the skin so staff are warned to protect themselves, Edna was not given any protection, her mouth was red raw and blistered, her tongue swollen and the tracks where the drug had run down her face were marked by scabs from too many burns. Edna was no longer able to feed herself so a power abuser lifted her head out of her uneaten food and poured liquid poison down her throat before dropping her head back on the plate. Edna became more dehydrated and malnourished as time went on and the drug concentrated even more in her system. Her eyes were crusted with discharge and her lips dark blue as she rasped, her eyes opened suddenly and I thought she recognised me because she put out her hand and gently rubbed my arm and I remembered a time not so long ago when a sprightly happy women had done the same. They had taken everything from Edna and they said it was alright, well it was not alright. Poor Edna after all she had suffered, could still stretch out her hand in trust to another even then, that one gesture was to dam them all because it was what I remembered whenever I was tired from the fight and wanted to give up, it was Edna's face that I remembered throughout all the hardship that was to follow. They thought her voice would never be heard but they feared Edna before long not because she shamed them but because she was a threat to what they valued most, their profit's.

It was May 1999, the investigation continued and so did the harassment, every hour you were in the building you were so afraid that it was a physical sickness you felt in your guts. There was only one thing worse than the hatred and harassment suffered the day before and that was the fear of what was yet to come. I did not know when the next chair would smash into me or if the constant threats of physical violence would be carried out. I had walked through the door to work hundreds of times, I never imagined that one day it would take everything I had to just go to work. It took more each time and I can honestly say that the prospect of climbing Everest would have looked like the easy option compared to walking through that wall of hate. I arrived to work a late shift and Maggie said there was a message in the book asking as many staff as possible from unit two attend Bill's funeral. Bill was one of our residents who had died in hospital, he had no relatives so it was normal practice in such circumstances for a request like this be made so I never questioned it or suspected anything and went about arranging extra staff to cover on the day of the funeral. I found out much later that the message was written on a "post it" note which was stuck in the message book and could just as easily be removed.

The day of Bill's funeral came and I had worked an on-call shift the night before and was working an early shift that morning. I had arranged for two staff to cover our absence and the other two unit's were fully staffed with the usual three staff on each. We did not have a break so when the two staff arrived to cover we left and stopped at the office on our way out. Big Maria was sitting there alone and we asked her if there were any flowers to take, she said they had been sent so we left in Maggie's car. Renee and Linda were going to the funeral before starting their late shift and were at the crematorium when we arrived, just as Bill's hearse drew up we were all surprised to see Carole Jones and Big Maria walk towards us, they never spoke to us and we all returned to Isard House afterwards. As soon as we walked through the door all hell broke loose. Rochelle who worked on unit three started screaming at us accusing us of leaving the home with no staff and walking out without permission. I was stunned by this and in spite of being surrounded by a mob who had turned up and who were screaming similar accusations. For the first time I shouted back. It was so blatantly untrue and I pointed out how many of them were surrounding me while their residents were the ones left unattended. Rochelle then changed the attack and said her unit was left with only two staff, but that was because she had deliberately sent the third member of staff to my unit when they had arrived. I had to shout to be heard and said," Why would you send your staff to this unit to give us three staff, when has this unit ever been given three staff?" I had tried to use reason but I knew it was no use as the mob had been whipped up to a frenzy and it did not matter that we had done nothing wrong. The rest of that shift was so bad I really do not know how we got through it. The mob walked up and down constantly, the dining room door was slammed so hard I thought the glass would shatter. Every time a door slammed we all flinched, Linda was trying to feed Aimee and they were both crying, the cleaners were stood behind shouting "Scum is what you are, scum." It all seemed to be happening in slow motion and as they shouted the abuse I noticed how their faces were all twisted, there mouths kept screaming "Scum, Scum" and the tears ran down Linda's face so slowly, God help us I kept saying over and over in my head, God help us.

It was may 13th 1999 and we all finished our shifts at the various times that day and went home, we were never to return, we made no conscious decision to leave it was more of a silent inevitable surrender to the fact we could not endure any more and needed to get help. I found out much later that Carole Jones had gone to get Dick Turner on some pretext that day so he would be at the front of the building when she pointed out we were leaving the home without permission and leaving residents with no staff. Thankfully it backfired because Mr Turner went to check and found all the unit's fully staffed. When he returned both Carole Jones and Big Maria had left the building and gone to the funeral in spite of the critical staff shortage they had alleged. They had used a resident's funeral as bait. It was never a consideration to them that Bill's death might have been a sad time for the staff who had long cared for him. It was just seen as another opportunity to fabricate evidence against us. We were the ones who were seen as the problem the abuse and abusers on the other hand were quite acceptable to them. In fact in our employer's eyes reporting abuse made us such bad people that on the day we were forced out of the home BUPA's senior management team came in with chocolates for every member of the mob in recognition of their services.

I rang Dick Turner that day when I got home and told him we needed help from someone higher up in BUPA. It was arranged that we should meet with BUPA Director, Des Kelly the next day, May 14th 1999. I rang Isard House and said two of us would not be able to work an early shift in full the next day as we were due to meet Mr Kelly and would have to leave early. I was halfway through explaining when Barbara, who was the on-call officer screamed abuse and put the phone down. I just started crying and Steve asked me what was wrong and I told him what had happened when I was trying to swap staff around so we could go and meet with Mr Kelly and get the help we so

desperately needed, Steve said, "Surely Mr Kelly could have got staff to cover from one of the five BUPA homes nearby. It seems to me they are deliberately making this as hard as possible for you to even ask for help."
I had been too tired to see it but he was right after all Mr Kelly knew why we wanted to meet with him but we were all so desperate to keep our jobs we did not see what was happening until we stood back from the nightmare situation we had endured for so long. All our strength had been taken up with finding a way to walk through the door of that home each day and bear the hell that our working lives had become. When I look back I really do not know how we lasted as long as we did.

It was well past midnight on May 13th before I had finished telephoning the six others, I told them that I had tried to cover our absence but it had been rejected and the phone banged down, we could not go on working in those conditions so we have to meet with Mr Kelly. I said I would ring Mr Turner in the morning and tell him we could not get cover. I could say no more as by this point I had been without sleep for thirty six hours straight having finished a twenty four hour shift some twelve hours earlier. The next morning I rang Dick Turner and told him what had happened when I tried to cover us to go to the meeting. I said we had two choices, either not meet Mr Kelly which meant we could not get help so would not be able to work or meet Mr Kelly, either way we could not work. Mr Turner said he understood the predicament we were in. The seven of us met two hours before the meeting with Mr Kelly was due to take place so we could prepare all the information we wanted him to have. We were all so desperate to keep our jobs that we knew this was our last chance to get help so we wanted to make sure he understood everything in full about what was happening to us and how it was making us ill.

The meeting took place at two o'clock at Durham house, the meeting was attended by myself and the other six carers. Dick Turner and Des Kelly and Monica Handscomb came in a little later. Mr Kelly spent some time telling us about his qualifications and the books he had written on social care. When he finished two of us did a presentation of all the facts to him. We had prepared a flip chart which listed all the staff on each unit in the home. We used coloured stickers next to the names of the staff who had abused the residents and a different colour sticker to separate the staff who were involved in the harassment. We talked about the abuse that had occurred and used four residents to demonstrate the kinds of abuse that had been inflicted. We then talked about going to Carole Jones and how we then had no choice but to go to Social Services. The largest part of the meeting was kept for the harassment which we detailed at great length and then each of us told him about what we had suffered individually. I felt moved by each of these accounts and really felt that Mr Kelly would act now that he knew what was happening. When we had finished speaking Mr Kelly said he took full responsibility and that he had not known we were being harassed and understood why we were all too sick to carry on working. He thought we should remain of sick until he got everything sorted out and then we could safely return to work. He said he would keep us informed of his progress and assured us that everything we had told him would be acted upon.

We never heard from Mr Kelly again, he later stated that he did not recall anything we had said, he did not even recall agreeing to meet with us. In fact the words "I do not recall" were to pretty much sum Mr Kelly up.
After that meeting the only contact I had from BUPA was a phone call from a hostile H.R women who demanded to know why I was not in work.

TWO

BEYOND ISARD HOUSE

God it would have been easy to walk away from it all then, but something inside told me that if I did it would be saying the abuse was alright, that it did not matter and I was wrong for reporting it to Social Services. It was not a matter of choice because I knew the abuse was wrong, so wrong that if I gave up now I would be as bad as those that committed the abuse and those who said it was alright. So I did the only thing I could do, I fought back and for the first time in my life I understood why other people fought for things when they could have had an easy life instead. There are some things we have to fight for if we do not than a part of us dies, the best part of us. We were all signed off work sick with stress, sometimes we got paid our statutory sick pay and sometimes we did not. "Oh you have only received £8.oo this month, we will pay what's short in next month's pay" we would be told by BUPA's wages Department, and it was all quite legal as they did pay it eventually but six weeks is a long time to survive on eight pounds. All of our family's were great and helped us but Lee could not pay his rent and had notice of eviction served on him. We sold everything we had of value at boot sales and when our possessions ran out then relatives and friends gave us their possessions to sell. The money we made would then be given to the one who was in most trouble that week. Some of the relatives from Isard House found out what had happened to us and gave us things to sell. After the story of the first court hearing hit the papers, total strangers sent us money, one of my greatest treasures is a card I received from a member of the public it said, "I am 84 years old so I can not afford to give you much but I sincerely hope you will accept the enclosed five pounds with my heartfelt gratitude, for what you did for those elderly people in Isard House, you did for me." The strange thing is that never in my life had I been so broke and yet never had I been so rich, I framed that card and it reminds me through the hard times that I will always be rich and that BUPAS two million a year chief executive, Val Gooding, will never be as rich as me. If anything I pity her for she had no reason for her absolute denial except a few billion in profit. I on the other hand had the best motivation of all to fight for, Edna, Dot, Grace, Jessie and all the others who touched my life and made it richer for knowing them, poor Val Gooding could never match that motivation.

Like most people in our situation we were certainly not in a position to pay for legal advice, we were lucky to just survive. There is no legal aid for Employment Tribunal cases. How very ironic that because you have lost your job, you have no money to access the laws protection when that's exactly why you need the laws protection in the

first place. Fortunately for us Linda knew a retired
barrister and she asked his advice. He said we
had to get legal representation urgently and gave
us details of a solicitor he knew personally. So we
made an appointment to see this solicitor and all
went to London to meet her, the name of the firm
was, Stephens Innocent, and we met with Sally
Gilbert and Sarah Culshaw. I always wondered
who Stephen was and what he was innocent of
and I meant to ask but there was so much to tell I
never got round to finding out. We told Sarah and
Sally everything that happened and that we were
off sick with stress and had been attending group
counselling for over a month, which Mr Turner had
arranged after the meeting on May 14th as he
could see that we were traumatised. They asked
us why our employer had not paid for or even
arranged counselling as it was their responsibility
not Social Services. It just had not occurred to us
to expect anything from our employers by that
point. They agreed to take our case on a no win,
no fee arrangement and said they would be writing
to Mr Kelly and asking him why he could not see
what Mr Turner had seen regarding our health and
ask what action he had taken to date to make it
safe for us to return to work. A while after this
letter was received by BUPA they then sent us all
details of a Telephone counselling service, which
came much too late for those of whose who had
their Telephones disconnected. We would not
have received even that pretence of help if we had
not obtained a solicitor. When there was no
response other then denial I did wonder if Mr Kelly

was the right person for our solicitor to be writing to. I had told Carole Newton and BUPA's H.R department about the harassment long before we were forced out of the building and they must have in turn informed Mr Kelly who did nothing to help us and now that we had a solicitor he was trying to cover-up his own failure to act, by continually denying he knew anything was wrong, as such his own conduct was questionable throughout.

I thought that if someone at the top of BUPA knew then they would be appalled at such events and would do something to help us, but I did need to know someone by name so asked Steve to ring BUPA House in London to ask them who the chairman was. He rung them and they said there were quite a few chairman, so we took the name of one immediately rang our solicitor and asked her to write to Sir Brian Nicholson and to tell him everything that had happened which she did. I was still trusting enough to believe that BUPA's senior management would be appalled at what had gone on, how could they not be I thought. However we later found out that BUPA Chief Executive, Val Gooding, C.B.E, had been informed of events in Isard House from the outset, had I known that at the time then I would not have been shocked at all by the letter of response we received from the BUPA Legal Department on behalf of Sir Brian Nicholson which made BUPA's stance clear. They believed Des Kelly's version of events of the meeting of May 14th, after all the trouble we went to get that meeting. It apparently slipped our minds to tell Mr Kelly about the harassment but we had just made some general reference to it in passing, and we had not given any names of the staff involved so they could not investigate it. We were all stunned by this response because it was so blatantly untrue. We knew nobody could have done more then us to ask for help. We had told Mr Kelly everything that was happening and went to all the trouble of making a detailed chart with the names of all those staff that were responsible written out for him as we thought it would help him in his investigations, which he took away with him. Our solicitor said she would keep trying to get them to investigate and in the meantime she would start proceedings in an Employment Tribunal as it took such a long time to be allocated a slot for a hearing. She duly informed BUPA of this and that we claimed the protection of The Public Interest Disclosure Act which had recently come into force and was to protect Whistle-blowers from harassment.

It was July 1999, Social Services had completed their inquiry and the report of their findings had been sent to BUPA's legal team to approve. The final report was published at the end of July and was the result of much negotiation with BUPA, when it should only have been the result of the available evidence, in spite of all BUPAS efforts the report was damning. We were not allowed to see a copy as BUPA had demanded it be kept confidential, but later due to BUPA's denial at our subsequent Tribunal hearing the report was made public and we saw it for the first time.

The report (Source Social Services Inquiry Report) listed all the abuse that was reported which included the following:

Hitting, Kicking, Spitting and punching residents, Verbal intimidation and restraint,
Withholding prescribed medication and overdosing using drugs that had not been authorised by the G.P,
Not calling G.Ps when medical emergencies were reported,
Neglect, lack of care, theft of belongings and financial abuse,
Failures of management to investigate and respond to incidents of abuse and neglect.

The inquiry conclusions are as follows,

"Although the witnessed incidents of physical abuse are not recent there is a significant number of witnesses amongst care staff employed in the home, relatives and others who have been interviewed and who corroborate the original allegations, a climate of complacency and laxness occurred in terms of the care of residents, inappropriate behaviour towards them did occur in the manner suggested by the witnesses who came forward and those subsequently interviewed."

"The outcome of this inquiry concludes that on unit three for a period between June 1998 and March 1999 a number of incidents occurred which were unacceptable in terms of the conduct of the staff and management of the welfare of residents, as such section nine of the Registered Care Homes Act 1984 has been breeched."

I asked what action the Police were going to take and eventually found out that no action was to be taken due to the crimes being out of date and secondly because the victims were not considered good witness's due to them suffering from dementia. The actions of Carole Jones amounted to perverting the course of justice as she had concealed the crimes that were now out of date and as for the residents dementia making them unsuitable witnesses it was the dementia that made them the victims of the crimes in the first place and now it was given as the reason why they could not have justice.

It was late August 1999, and the phone rings at five a.m. and I jump out of bed to answer it. It is Lee who has been up all night waiting for a reasonable time to ring me and gave up and could wait no longer, when he told me why I could understand. He told that the night before his friend had treated him to a night out at the pub as he had no money for a long time and his friend thought it would cheer him up, whilst at the pub. Later in the evening a care worker from another care home recognised Lee from a course they had both attended so came over for a chat. It was just by chance that this carer mentioned that one of the senior staff from Isard House was due to start work at another BUPA care home nearby. When Lee asked for the name of the staff member, he was horrified to be told it was Maria Keenahan. I was stunned and asked Lee if he was sure and he said Little Maria was due to start work next Tuesday which was the day after the August Bank Holiday, I told Lee I would meet him at Bromley South train station at eight thirty and we would then go to Bromley Social Services together. As I got ready to meet Lee my mind was churning, had we been lied to all along and misplaced our trust in Dick Turner? Did he know about this all along and only told us the inquiry report upheld the allegations to get rid of us? If not then why were BUPA able to ignore the report? The questions went round and round in my head.

When Lee and I arrived at the civic centre I was determined to get these questions answered, as soon as I told Dick Turner about Little Maria I knew from the look of shock on his face that he had not known. He said he would find out if it were true and he promised us that he would never allow Maria to work with vulnerable people again and that he had made this very clear to BUPA. He asked for some time to check it out and said he would ring later. Dick Turner rang the next morning and said it was true and that he had rung Mr Kelly and told him it was out of the question, the name of that care home was Anne Sutherland

House.

The summer of 1999 continued to pass and we were told that Carole Jones had resigned and moved to Shropshire. Big Maria left to work elsewhere and Sarah and little Maria remained suspended, we were told. The fact that BUPA had tried to place Little Maria in another of their care homes had shaken us all to the core. We just could not understand why they would let her near elderly people when they knew what she had done and was capable of doing again. A while later we were told Sarah had resigned but were unable to find out if she would be given references by BUPA if she applied for another care job. Little Maria remained suspended and we could not understand why she had not been sacked. We decided that we should visit our MPs but it being late summer most were away on holiday. Our first appointment was with one of their aides and we all travelled to London so excited that we even had a photograph taken to mark the occasion. In the photograph we are all standing on the green, the Houses of Parliament behind us. We all looked so confident and were convinced that nothing could matter more then our residents to those that sat in the house behind us. Then we walked into the House of Commons Lobby and waited in awed silence for the aide to meet us. A short while later he appeared and introduced himself. He seemed to be very nice. He escorted us across the road to his office and as we walked I could not help staring at the hems on his trousers which had both

come undone and had been for sometime by the
look of them, both his shoe heels where covered
by the threadbare remains of the material, which
was the only reason he did not constantly trip and
only occasionally stumbled. We reached the
building on the other side of a busy street and we
all entered one at a time through glass tubes that
looked like something from the Star ship
Enterprise. We followed him to a lift which took us
to an office several floors up. He showed us in and
said he would be right back. We all stared around
the cramped room and I wondered how they
managed to get so much stuff into such a small
space, there were papers stacked on top of the
filing cabinets that reached to the ceiling, every
surface was piled with folders and papers even
the windowsills. Lee picked up an envelope from a
pile nearby, "Look it's got the House of Commons
on it." We all looked at it with interest impressed at
how important it looked. I did not know then that
hundreds of those envelopes would routinely
come through my letter box every month. The aide
came back with several plastic boxes for us to sit
on and we all sat down. He looked genuinely
shocked when we told him what had happened
and every now and then would say something
usually "Good Lord that surely can not be legal.
"When we finally finished he said the whole thing
was a disgrace and that he would be contacting
his boss immediately. He then escorted us out of
the building and this time we took the stairs so he
could point out all the paintings that hung on the
walls, he would stop at each painting and give us

an account of the sitter and artist, when we arrived at an empty space on the wall he turned and said "Oh dear now where has that got to?" As if we could provide the answer, he said he would go and find out and he left us standing there on the stairs for a couple of minutes, he returned and announced that the painting had gone to be cleaned and we all nodded then moved on.

When we finally arrived downstairs he assured us that we would hear from him soon. We said goodbye and all entered the glass tubes one at a time and were all gathered on the pavement outside when the aide seemed to have forgotten something and entered a glass tube pointing. He got stuck and after much pulling and pushing at his glass container he seemed to resign himself to his fate and started pointing again and shouted "I wanted to tell you the train station is that way" and we all smiled and nodded and walked off. I looked back once and he was still there pushing at the glass, oh my God I thought these people are running the country. Don't get me wrong he was a very nice man, I just had no idea people like that existed except in, Poirot or Jeeves stories, not in the real world. We all walked along lost in our own thoughts for a while, our silence only broken when Renee said suddenly "Did you see the state of his bleeding trousers? "We all laughed.

Steve had a word processor which he used occasionally to make headings for his paintings. I remember the first time I used it, it had taken me all day to write a long letter and I was almost finished when it all disappeared of the screen. Steve came into the room to see I why I was running around in a panic. He just hit a button and it all came back and I was so relieved as I thought it was all lost. It was a letter to the Secretary of State for Health, which at the time was Frank Dobson. I was writing to him because even though Isard House was managed by BUPA under contract, it was owned by Bromley Council, which had contracted out all its six Care Homes to BUPA. I did not realise then that in writing that letter I was making what the law calls, "Qualifying Disclosures." That was the first letter of several hundred written that first year but it must have had some impact because a team came down from The Department of Health and copied all the files on our case.

Meanwhile BUPA continued with the stance that they could not investigate our concerns as they were not aware we had any. No one could have possibly done more in asking for help before we were forced out of the building and since. I had met with Carole Newton twice and the H.R department and still nothing was done, yet we had still found the trust to go to a more senior BUPA manager, Des Kelly and when still nothing is done I like a fool hold onto a shred of hope that someone at the top of this company will help us and ask that an appeal be made to Sir Brian Nicholson who also fails to help us. God either the managers, Directors, Chairman and H.R

Department of the company are all suffering from the worst case of memory loss ever recorded, or there's a culture of, cover-up and Deny at any cost, so ingrained in this company it's from the top down, as the first explanation defied medical science I could only presume it was the later. We had up to this point only seen a glimpse of the cover-up culture, what was to follow was beyond anything we had seen so far. The first starve out tactic now began, BUPA offered to meet with each of us one at a time. They knew full well we could not afford to have a solicitor present over seven separate meetings. We continued to offer to meet as a group and could not understand why they refused this, our solicitor then explained all, "it's a common starve out tactic used against people like yourselves with limited legal resources. Do not worry it's so common that it will be obvious to any court what they are doing", she told us. I felt uneasy about that and thought what kind of legal system would allow such a terrible thing as starving people out to be used to the point it has become common?

It was November 1999 and we all faced the prospect of a very bleak Christmas. One morning Lee rang me and when I heard his voice my heart sunk. He said that Maria Keenahan has been working in another BUPA care home called Faircroft, which is in Penge. I asked him if he was sure and he said the person who told him was trustworthy but he had promised not to reveal their name, "You know what BUPA do to staff who say anything", he said and I promised him he would not have to reveal his source and that I would not say where I had got the information but would go straight to Dick Turner, I told Lee I would ring him when I got some news. I set off for Bromley and by the time I reached the Civic centre my heart was pounding and I had gone over everything a hundred times, when Dick Turner appeared I realised how angry I had become as I shouted at him, "Is Maria Keenahan working?" I watched his face closely and he was shocked when he replied "It is impossible BUPA knows she is a grave danger and that has been made abundantly clear to them. "I told him that I had it on good authority that she is working at Faircroft care home and in a much quieter voice he said" She can not be. "I told him that I believed she was and shouted" I have seen what that woman is capable of doing, how could she be let near defenceless elderly people to do it again, I do not know who to trust anymore. It seems to me that BUPA are doing what they like, why aren't they listening?" I shouted, I felt more then anger it was sheer frustration that after all we had done to stop this women she was still free to abuse more people.

Dick Turner stood there in silence listening and when I finished he said he could understand how I felt and if it were true I had every right to feel that way. He asked me to give him a short time to investigate "it must be a mistake", he said and promised to call me later that day. I agreed reluctantly and went home to wait. I could not understand what was happening. I had always thought that if Social Services said an abuser could not work than that would be good enough for any care company but BUPA knew what Maria was capable of and they don't care who she hurts. Later that day Dick Turner rang me and for a moment I did not recognise the quite voice that said," It's true she was working there but will not be anymore." There was a long silence and he asked me if I could hear him, I said I heard him but I just did not know what to say. What happens next? I asked him after a few minutes, he said there would be an investigation and he would keep me informed of what happened. I dreaded telling the others I knew how sick it would make them feel.

It was around Christmas 1999 when Dick Turner rang and said that when he had rung Des Kelly in August to stop Little Maria from working at Anne Sutherland care home, Mr Kelly agreed she could not work, but the day after he sent her to work at Faircroft instead, which was down the road from Anne Sutherland House. Little Maria had worked there since. We all made the decision to resign that day and we all did so within a short time once our letters of resignation had been approved by our solicitor. I resigned because I could not work for a company who would knowingly turn a blind eye to such abuse and who would dam anyone who was not willing to do the same.
We all had kept the hope we would be able to keep our jobs but it was impossible to go back.

Without any investigation into the harassment there was no accountability, the staff had BUPA's full approval to harass us and to have gone back would have been to suffer even worse treatment. I wanted to go to the press then. I told the solicitor it was the only way to stop BUPA sending Little Maria into another care home to abuse, "You have to trust in the law", she told me. We did trust in the law but we had to wait for the law to hear us and while we waited BUPA could hide Little Maria in yet another care home and the possibility that she could be left alone behind closed doors with yet another vulnerable resident, was just too much to bear. We decided if we could not go to the press, then we would have to watch the homes ourselves. Between us we managed to scrounge two pairs of Binoculars, a camera and a thermos flask which we kept in what became known as the "Surveillance bag."
We would pick one of the six BUPA care homes in the area and then watch it for a fortnight before moving on to the next home, we drew up a rota and took it in turns to stand watch.

One night not long after this Karen and I were watching Faircroft it was late so it was dark and we sat in the car with the engine turned off so as not to attract any attention. It was freezing cold and we were shivering so much at times I could hardly hold a cup of tea without spilling it. We waited for the late shift to finish so did not expect any movement by the front door. So when we saw someone by the door it immediately drew our attention, through the glass front door of the home we saw two residents briefly in the hallway. They tried to open the door and then they turned and walked off arm in arm, Karen and I both immediately said, "Rose and Jessie" simultaneously, it was in a way like touching base, a quick sharp reminder that we had not gone totally mad and were sitting there for a good reason. Another night a while later I was sitting watching a different home when I suddenly thought what in God's name are we doing here. Who would ever have thought we would have to go to such lengths to stop abuse. We kept up the surveillance right up to the time we had to go to court and then we resumed it after the hearing, our perseverance paid off and subsequently we discovered Little Maria working in two more BUPA care homes.

Our case at the Employment Tribunal was to be heard at Ashford and we were finally allocated dates for a hearing, which would take place in July 2000. Our solicitor found a barrister willing to take our case on in spite of the fee being paid in instalments, his name was Ian Scott from Old Square Chambers and we all liked him, he was very confident about our case and kept saying "You are the perfect Whistle-blowers and have done all that the law has asked of you." Our solicitor said we needed to start preparing our witness statements early as the procedure for "Exchanging the bundles" would formally take place a while before the hearing and once all the evidence had been exchanged we could not add anything we had forgotten when we saw it in BUPAS statements, she explained changing statements would not make us credible witness's in the eyes of the Tribunal and the other side would make sure the Tribunal knew about it. I could understand why that was the procedure but none of us were in the least bit worried about our statements as we were always telling the truth so had nothing to fear. So we all began writing our statements and once I had finished mine I sent it to the solicitor Sarah Culshaw, who said it was miles too long and I would have to cut it by three quarters, "but I wont be able to get it all in", I said to her. She said that BUPA did not dispute the abuse in their formal court response, well how could they dispute that I thought when it has been upheld by the Authorities, she went on to say that our harassment was fully disputed and I should concentrate on getting that in my statement, she said we could use a few examples of the abuse but only as background information and the rest should be about harassment. We all found this a very hard thing to do as the abuse was so tied up in everything, it took me at least five or six drafts before the solicitor accepted my statement and only then grudgingly as she still thought it much too long, thank God we all dug our heels in about the examples of abuse we insisted be kept in, most of all thank God that I kept Edna's abuse in mine.

Linda met one of the relatives from Isard house in

the High Street one day and they exchanged
telephone numbers and addresses, the relative
then sent Linda a copy of a Isard House
newsletter which had been given to all the
relatives and which proudly announced who would
be replacing myself and Maggie as team leader
and senior on unit two, only this announcement
was made two months before Maggie and I had
even resigned, which was not as shocking as who
was chosen to take our jobs, Anne Davidson who
had smashed a chair into my back was promoted
to senior and Nadeen was promoted to team
leader, these are the kind of people BUPA want,
abusers and their supporters not people like
myself and Maggie who were trouble makers
because we reported abuse. Dick Turner was sent
a copy of the newsletter but we were still not sure
if we could trust him as BUPA could do what they
wanted. We continued to prepare for the Tribunal,
BUPA asked for our interview notes with Social
Services which we were never shown and when
we received them we told Dick Turner that more
then half of them were missing, no doubt taken by
the Health Department we thought. Then there
was an almighty fuss made by BUPA who did not
want to be called BUPA in the court paperwork
and wanted to be called, Care First, I said to the
solicitor Sarah that there is a huge blue and white
sign outside Isard House and it clearly says,
"BUPA" and it makes no mention of Care First and
our contracts of employment led us to believe we
worked for BUPA, the fuss went on and on and to
our dismay Sarah Culshaw gave in under the

pressure. I thought it was a great shame that BUPA could put such a huge effort into protecting their name and reputation when they had not lifted a finger to protect those residents in their care.

Not long before the case was due to start Sarah Culshaw and Sally Gilbert went to work for a new law firm called, Bolt Burden and Sarah Culshaw was now made the lead solicitor on our case and Sally Gilbert oversaw things occasionally. Sarah Culshaw asked Dick Turner if he would write a statement about the events he had witnessed and he agreed. We did not expect him to tell the truth as we were not as trusting as we once had been, due to the missing witness statements and BUPA doing what they liked. We all felt really terrible when we saw his statement, as he had told the whole truth and we knew how hard it was to do that when BUPA were involved, Dick Turners statement was damming and he was now a threat to BUPA's reputation and they preserved their reputation at all costs. Linda pretty much summed up the situation Dick Turner was now in, once she read his statement she said, "Poor sod is in for it now."

Before our case began Sarah Culshaw suggested we go down to the Ashford Employment Tribunal and sit on another case so we got familiar with how everything worked. We went to Ashford one day shortly afterwards, the Employment Tribunal was in Tuften Street opposite the Magistrates Court, the exterior of the Tribunal gave no clue as to it's activities it just looked like a office block. We told the clerk who answered the intercom that we wanted to sit in the public area, he came down and unlocked the door and took us to a large empty room, "The case will Start in a minute" he told us and went to stand by the door. I looked around the room, it was very large with a high ceiling and on one side two large windows took up almost the whole wall. I was sitting in the back row of four long rows of seats, directly in front of these were two long tables, one for each side's legal team I presumed. Then of to the right the blue carpeted floor had a wooden square on which stood a small table and chair, this was the area known as "The Stand "or witness box in the more traditional courts. The most prominent feature in the whole room ran the length of the wall opposite, a long wooden bench several feet high allowing those who sat behind it to look down on the room in exactly the same way as a judge in any other court would. This bench is where the Tribunal panel would sit, three people in all, two lay members who were not legally qualified and the third person was the chairman who was usually a solicitor qualified in employment law and who had the final say.

The case began and several people came in through the door held open by the clerk, then the three members of the panel came through a door behind the bench and we all stood up until the panel were seated. The case seemed to be in the final stages so it was hard to grasp what it was all about, there was a lot of legal jargon and it all sounded very complicated, everything was conducted very formally in the same way it would be in any other Court. We sat and listened all morning and then they adjourned for lunch and we left none the wiser as to what the case was about, but at least we knew what to expect and how to find the place next time. We stood outside the Tribunal for a short time discussing what we had seen and heard, but we quickly moved on for it was cold despite being a warm spring day. We discovered later it was always cold there, the wind howled around the Tribunal building which was in the permanent shadow of the much larger court opposite, it was a grey and dismal place to have to spend any amount of time in, we were to spend far too much time there before the case was over. A directions hearing date was allocated before the case was heard in full, Sarah Culshaw explained it was special time set aside to hear all legal arguments. That meant that the time allocated for the case would be to hear the evidence as all the legal arguments would have already been dealt with. I thought this seemed a good idea as we had already waited over a year to have our evidence heard and we were all desperate to read our statements. We went down to the directions hearing and saw the panel who would be judging our case for the first time, the first of the lay members was a short thickset man with white hair and a very red face, his name was Mr T.J. Lane, The other lay member was a women in her fifties who was very smartly dressed and looked quite stern, her name was Mrs Greenman, then there was the chairman who sat in the centre, his name was Mr M. Zuke, he was a solicitor whose area of expertise was employment law, he was small and thin with an impassive face and rarely spoke that day.

I suppose we had all expected BUPA to have only one barrister and a solicitor like ourselves, we did not expect to see an army which filled over half the seats behind their two barristers, the first of which was Laura Cox Q.C, who was a small blond women in her fifties and who was extremely intimidating and rather bossy, next to her sat Mr Paul Epstein, who looked far too experienced to be a mere junior, we discovered that the army behind them consisted of solicitors from BUPA's large in house Legal Department, a press relations team of spin doctors and most of the BUPA H.R Department. I took notes and listened intently to the heated legal arguments that went on all day, the main thrust of BUPA's defence seemed to be that, we were such complete and utter liars and that our case should not even be heard at all, they called us "Vexatious" and "Frivolous" quite a lot and it was just as well I did not know what that meant until I looked the words up in the dictionary when I got home that night. In short BUPA said we were bringing the case against them out of spite and that we had not a shred of evidence to support the fact we were telling the truth. I felt really angry at first but I quickly realised it was a pretty poor defence when you considered all the evidence we had to support our version of events and independent evidence at that. After the directions hearing was over Ian Scott our barrister said he thought it had gone very well, "Trust in the law you are the perfect Whistle-blowers and the law will protect you" he said before we all left. We all looked forward to the hearing, for us it was the light at the end of the tunnel that we all clung to, the prospect that what had started when we reported the abuse more then a year ago, would soon be over and we could get on with our lives. The hearing was to start on July 10th 2000 and was allocated six full days which was plenty of time to hear all the evidence now that the legal arguments had all been dealt with.

None of us had gone into court for money it was not about that, we could see no other way of bringing BUPA to account and unless that happened then BUPA would continue to deny the abuse and employ Little Maria. We wanted justice for ourselves but also for the residents we had tried to protect, and whilst we accepted that a Tribunal was not the criminal trial that should have happened, it was the only justice we had access to.

The bundles were exchanged and each side had plenty of time to read the other sides evidence and prepare for cross examination, but when we saw BUPA's evidence for the first time we could not have been more shocked, of course we were prepared for them to dispute that we had been harassed, it was what we had expected and had prepared our case for. But we never imagined they would equally deny the abuse, they said we had made it all up, which was incredible given it was upheld to be true and all the available evidence supported it to be true. BUPA's culture of denial knew no limit's. Sarah Culshaw and Ian Scott saw BUPA's stance of total denial as the advantage it was in reality and they both told us not to worry about it as in denying the abuse which had been proven to be true and was fully upheld by the authorities, then BUPA's denial of the harassment detracted from their credibility. We counted the days until the hearing and at last it was time, we arrived at the Ashford Tribunal early that first day and we were shown into a room with a sign on the door reading, applicants, BUPA had their own waiting room further down the hall. Ian Scott our barrister was already there and explained that I was to be called first and would read my statement out and then be cross-examined until around lunchtime and then Maggie would be called next and so on.

We were called by the clerk and we all trooped into the court room, followed by BUPA's large crowd. I sat gripping my witness statement in anticipation and waited to be called to the stand, as we were supposed to be putting our case first we were surprised when Laura Cox Q.C stood up and proceeded to argue what were legal points that should have been raised in the earlier directions hearing. I sat there watching the clock show first the minutes and then the hours tick by and then prospect that the evidence may not all be heard in the time that remained occurred to me for the first time. When we adjourned for lunch I asked Ian Scott what would happen if we ran out of time and he said the case would go part heard and we would have to wait for new dates to be allocated.

After Lunch Laura Cox continued with her legal arguments and as the time ticked by I feared we would lose a whole day and then suddenly it got even worse, Laura Cox said she was going to appeal and the Tribunal was adjourned for two whole days whilst the appeal was heard in London.

We were all devastated but Ian Scott and Sarah Culshaw said we should not worry it was just a starvation tactic to delay the case and that there would still be time for all our evidence to be heard. We went home with heavy hearts as there was no longer any end in sight, it seemed we would have to wait ages for the verdict which would prove we were telling the truth. This was so important to us as it would stop BUPA calling us liars publicly, BUPA made the first of two appeals, the second of which was reported in the media. Such appeals are known as starvation tactics as they delay the case, they have no other purpose.

Beyond The Facade

THE GUARDIAN LAW REPORT
10/11/00

"The Claimants brought proceedings against their employer claiming victimisation contrary to sections 44 and 47b of ERA, on the morning of the hearing before the Tribunal before the claimants opened their case and called their evidence, the employer made an application to strike out the case on the basis that even if all the evidence in the claimants witness statements were accepted as factually correct their claims could not proceed whether as a matter of fact or law or both"

BUPA's grounds for appeal pretty much summed up their attitude towards us from the start, they did not care if the residents were abused and they did not care that they were harassed, the only thing they cared about was their reputation. The ingrained culture of cover-up and deny at any cost included twisting the law to aide them in silencing us, BUPA did lose both of these appeals but succeeded in delaying the case. As far as I was concerned the law should never have allowed such a vexatious appeal in the first place. We returned to the Tribunal resigned to fact the case would go part heard, with only four of the allocated days left I was acutely aware of making the most of the time we had left and that as many of us as possible should read their statements. I was in such a rush when I read my statement that I had to be asked to slow down, even when I got to the sections of the statement that I knew would be upsetting as they were about the residents, I refused to have a break looking at the clock and knowing how desperate the others were to have their chance of putting the truth. When I had finished reading the statement Laura Cox Q.C commenced her cross examination and at times I got angry and frustrated with her questions but it got her nowhere as I had always told the truth she could not twist the truth no matter how hard she tried. I recall her accusing me of selling my story to the press and said "Do you mean for Money?" When she said yes, I replied, "There have certainly been times when we have had little food or money to buy it, but I can assure you that at no time would we ever take money for our story, in fact if I had the money I would pay the press to print it if that's what it takes to stop BUPA employing known abusers" and so it went on all morning until we adjourned for lunch.

After lunch I noticed Maggie sitting there gripping her statement waiting to be called but still my cross examination continued all of that day then the next, in all four whole days and then we ran out of time for the others to be heard at all.

Finally Laura Cox asked me a question and I answered and waited for the next question but she turned her back on me and started reading something, after about five minutes the chairman asked her if she had finished,"Yes" she snapped sharply.

I left the stand exhausted but happy. I still can not remember all the questions she asked me as sometimes they were so ridiculous it was obvious she was trying to waste time, but I had told the truth and that could not be twisted.

When I left the stand I did feel emotionally exhausted as it was people's lives that were at the centre of the case, we had not reported faulty machinery but the suffering of people we knew like family. As I left the court room one of the press who had been there throughout said to me "God I haven't seen a cross examination that long even at an Old Bailey murder trial" I smiled and thought to myself that BUPA would have me in the dock of The Old Bailey if they could make telling on them a crime. We had waited over a year for this hearing and we were all bitterly disappointed when it went part heard. We sat there waiting for new dates to be allocated, but when Ian Scott was available, then Laura Cox was not and when both were available then the Tribunal panel was not. We listened dismayed as the months were ticked off until finally a new hearing date was set, it was for the following March which meant seven whole months of waiting, which seemed for ever when we had waited so long already. The only consolation was in spite of the huge efforts by BUPA to suppress the evidence, at least my statement had been read and was now in the public domain and could be reported in the press.

Eileen Chubb

The Express (23/8/00)

GOVERNMENT ADVISOR AT CENTRE OF BUPA HOME ABUSE CASE.
By Lucy Johnson.

A Government advisor on care of the elderly is at the centre of allegations of widespread neglect at a residential home.

Des Kelly is one of the BUPA Directors responsible for 65-bed Isard House in Bromley Kent, where former staff say elderly residents were subjected to a shocking regime of abuse. Former staff claim they saw patients kicked, spat and screamed at, have their drugs withheld or be overdosed on tranquillisers and left lying in urine-soaked beds, they say that despite complaining to the homes managers for more than a year, no apparent action was taken until they reported their concerns to Kent Social Services, which called in Police.

The group is bringing a landmark claim for unfair dismissal under the 1998 Public Interest Disclosure Act. This offers protection to employees who come forward with evidence of malpractice or criminal activity.

Yesterday, David Hinchliff, chairman of the Commons Health Select Committee, said he was "Deeply concerned" by the allegations "This is extremely worrying, BUPA need to open up this whole case and make it public" he said" A company should never employ people to look after

*vulnerable people when there are such grave
questions over them and an investigation pending"
The news will also alarm Health Secretary Alan
Millburn, who recently praised the way BUPA was
working with the overstretched N.H.S. Graham
Smith, BUPA Care Services managing director
strongly denies the allegations.*

THE DAILY EXPRESS, EDITORIAL.

*We reveal today a horrifying story of neglect and
abuse at the privately run Isard House care home,
such stories are always deeply shocking, but what
makes this one especially so are the allegations
about the attitude of the owner, BUPA, the largest
private health and geriatric care company in the
country. It failed to take note of these claims or act
to make sure the culprit's were brought to book,
even worse it re-employed an alleged abuser in
another home, BUPA contests these allegations.
Most residential care for the elderly is provided in
private homes the greater part of it at the very
least is adequate, some much better than that, it
used to be the old council run homes were more
often and not a problem, but there is a unpleasant
undertone running through too many private
homes, which make all sorts of promises about
the standard of care they offer but which when
confronted with evidence to the contrary, simply
do not seem to listen to the employees on the
ground. BUPA makes precisely these promises,
indeed so fine is it's reputation that one of it's*

Directors, Des Kelly, has advised the Government. Yet our investigation reveals a profoundly worrying culture which runs throughout the company from bottom to top.
BUPA must act swiftly to ensure its employees procedures are models of good practice. If it continues to behave with such apparent contempt towards its Whistle-blowers the company will find it's self at the centre of a national scandal which could deservedly destroy its entire market.

This first story in the Express was important to us because it made the waiting more bearable, we were foolish enough to believe that it would finally stop BUPA hiding Little Maria in any more care homes, we were wrong which is hardly surprising when you consider the items on the BUPA list of denial so far.

1. The seven care staff who blew the whistle on the abuse, BUPA says, they are complete liars, there was never any abuse.

2. The medication records that prove drugs were withheld and intentionally illegally stockpiled in order to intentionally administer unauthorised doses in potentially lethal levels, BUPA say are also lying as there was no abuse.

3. The independent Pharmacist who said drugs were not given that should have been, that drugs

were not returned so are not accounted for and that tranquillisers were administered in amounts Maria Keenahan decided, BUPA say these medical records are lying as there was no abuse.

4. The twenty others who witnessed abuse also, including relatives, other staff and visitors, BUPA say are liars as there was no abuse.

5. The entire Social Services inquiry team who investigated and upheld the abuse, BUPA say are liars as there was no abuse.

In hindsight I realise that BUPA would have denied the abuse even if I had acquired the services of an independent camera man to film it, BUPA would just say the camera had lied. I could not have got BUPA to accept the abuse even had I employed the combined services of, Panorama, Kate Adie and Quentin Tarintino to present it to them, not even a witness list that included the Pope, Arch Bishop of Canterbury and the entire population of Greater London would have made them accept the abuse. BUPA would still deny it, they would deny it because they always knew it was true and with every day of denial that passed, the more they were implicated in the cover-up and the clock is still ticking.

What happened in Isard House was so acceptable to BUPA that they had no problem denying it, it is still acceptable to them today, all that suffering, pain and torture can be excused, I do wonder what BUPA would judge to be unacceptable, it would have to be something of biblical proportions and even then someone would have to tell, and who would dare do that?

We all had problems finding work, for example I would see a job advertised and ring up for an interview and as soon as I said my name there would be a silence before the question "Are you one of them BUPA people?" and I would be told the job had suddenly been filled even though it continued to be advertised. Some of us even kept quite about being a Whistle-blower as if reporting abuse was something we should feel ashamed of. It always caught up with you and sooner or later you would walk into the staff room and hear the dreaded whisper, "Whistle-blower."

Then there was the problem of getting time off for the Tribunal hearings, you never had enough holiday time and had to explain why you needed to have unpaid time off, as soon as you said why, you would see the suspicion in their eyes. We endured it and again and again. We counted the days to the hearing.

Finally it was March 2001 and the hearing was due to start at Ashford on March 5th and last for three and a half weeks. None of us had any holiday pay so we all had to survive a month with no money. Two of us had to choose between keeping our jobs or taking time off for court, so did not even have jobs to go back to. That's the result of starvation tactics, the harsh reality of surviving the legal process is you are entirely unprotected by the law while you seek its protection.

We pooled all the money we had managed to put by and using two cars just managed to cover the cost of the petrol to get us and there and back each day. There was no money left for food or even a cup of tea, so we all took packed lunches which consisted of a meagre amount to last twelve hours, BUPA will never know how close they came to starving us out literally as we all lost over a stone in weight.

The first day of the hearing began and we all trooped back into the court, Laura Cox Q.C stood up yet again and we all closed our eyes and prayed, not again, not when we had sacrificed so much to get there, but she only submitted three new witness statements which belonged to, Des Kelly, Carole Newton and Carole Jones.
Ian Scot made objections but the statements were accepted, so Ian Scott asked for a break in order to read them and we went back to the waiting room. I asked him how BUPA could be allowed to do that and he said "Do not worry they have now lost all credibility in the eyes of the Tribunal" so we all read the statements and it did not take long to see what had changed, they now attacked Dick Turner as they had read his statement. I thought Ian Scott was right as BUPA now looked just what they were, total liars who tried to silence anyone who dared tell the truth.

So the evidence began, our case was put first, I did find the hardest part was watching the others being cross examined, they were put through hell by BUPA for doing the right thing. They were all amazing and it was obvious they were telling the truth.

Maggie was called and read her statement and then was cross examined, she was accused of working on a Bromley market Stall when she was off sick, she was so mad she went down to the market and got statements from all the stall holders who confirmed they had never set eyes on her. Ian Scott went mad about it and it was only one of the two occasions I ever saw him lose his temper, he stood up and said to the panel,

"This is a very serious matter, they have accused this women of committing fraud in open court and have done so in spite of the fact there is not a shred of evidence to support such an accusation"
The chairman Mr Zuke agreed and told BUPA so.

Then Laura Cox put it to Maggie, that she had never told Des Kelly she was being harassed when she met with him, Maggie said, "We all told that man we were being harassed. He was told about all of it and Mr Turner was there and heard us tell him and he (Pointing at Des Kelly) is a complete liar for saying otherwise but we all told him alright and we can prove we did." Laura Cox had no more questions for Maggie after that and we went out for lunch, we sat on the car park wall and ate our sandwiches, "I could really murder a bag of chips now" said Maggie and we all looked at our sandwiches and sighed. I watched as each in turn took the stand and be cross examined by the very best that money could buy, I saw in each of them the unwavering certainty that comes only with the truth, the truth shone out of them and no matter what Laura Cox Q.C threw at it, she could not dim it, it's there for all to see in the unblinking eyes, the whole body language, you can not mistake it nor can you fake it, you would make a fortune if you could bottle it for politicians would queue up to buy it.

I remember how very young Lizzy looked when she took the stand, this tiny girl almost obscured from view by the piles of evidence on the table before her. She spoke out loud and clear and told of the terrible abuse she had seen and how frightened and alone she had felt, but still risked everything and went to report it to Carole Jones who had responded by shouting, "I will not have the word abuse said in my home." Carole had told Little Maria, who made Lizzy's life hell and locked her in the kitchen and threatened her. Lizzy then said she had to report the abuse to Social Services and how she was then harassed and when she could take no more went to Des Kelly and told him. When Laura Cox tryed to say that Des Kelly had only been told about the abuse Lizzy replied "Why would we tell him about that when we knew Social services were investigating it, we told him about some of the abuse only so he understood why we had gone to Social Services, we met him to report the harassment, why would we ask for a meeting to get help and then not tell him why we needed help? He must be deaf no one could have forgotten what we told him." Laura Cox had no further questions for Lizzie after that.

Lee being one of only three males at the hearing, was lucky not to have to queue up for the toilet, the Tribunal had only one cubical in the cramped ladies toilet and we all dreaded being in there with Laura Cox or one of the other female members of the large BUPA entourage. I ran in to use the toilet one day with Renee and it was empty, Renee waited and I called out to her from the cubical, when the last intact pair of knickers I had suddenly tore, I thought it was strange when she did not say anything in response as the state of our threadbare underwear was something we always tried to laugh at simply because we would have cried otherwise, when I came out of the cubical most of BUPAS legal team was standing there and looked suitable guilty being responsible for our underwear dilemmas, which I suppose also fell under starvation tactics. When I got outside I found Renee down the hall "Well I was not staying quashed up in there with them", she said. Karen, Linda, Lee and Renee had all given their evidence and our last witness was Dick Turner, who read his statement and was then cross examined, it quickly became apparent from the line of questioning that BUPA had decided to dispute the inquiry report they received two years earlier, for the first time. Again no matter what Laura Cox threw at it, it did not change the fact that the abuse had been upheld because it was true. Laura Cox then tried to discredit the inquiry report instead and this proved a mistake as it was formally submitted in evidence along with stacks of evidence in support of it's findings, such as the statements of other witness's, letters of complaint written about the lack of care at Isard House, the formal minutes of meetings with BUPA taken by the council clerk, which proved beyond doubt BUPA's evidence to be completely untrue to the point it would have been perjury in any other court of law. There were no further questions for Mr Turner after that. Finally it was time for BUPA to call their witness's who would then be cross examined by our barrister. Each evening I prepared a list of questions for Ian Scott to ask next day, at first he said "Don't you trust me?" but then after reading the list would say you have raised some important points here. Every morning I would arrive and hand over my list and it became so much part of the daily routine that if I arrived in the morning and did not give him a list he would ask if I had forgotten but I never did. No one knew the evidence better then we did because we had lived it, we also knew the witness's better then anyone and I tried to prepare Ian Scott for Maria Keenahan who was to be cross examined the next day. I told him about her personality and how she was likely to change her story that many times it would make him dizzy just trying to keep up with her twists and turns. I told him what a good actress she was and all the roles she could play and that I thought she would most likely play the idiot if cornered. Ian Scott listened to everything I told him and then said" I have dealt with much worse than her."

The next day when we were called into court, Maria Keenahan took the stand, when I saw her walk into the court room my stomach somersaulted and I felt the familiar sick dread she always invoked in me. The cross examination began and she never gave the same answer twice but constantly ducked and dived, she played the idiot as I had thought she would if cornered and said "Oh dear I am such a fool "constantly.
Ian Scott was good and did corner her and then a glimpse of what lay beneath the smiling mask would be revealed for a split second and her face would completely contort with rage, the contrast emphasised even more by how swiftly she regained the smiling mask. Nearly all of the cross examination was taken up with Edna's medication records and line by line sheet by sheet she confirmed it was her signature next to each of the illegal doses. She did her best to avoid this but the evidence was too much for her in the end but she still spun such a web that she made herself dizzy with it in the end. If she had a shred of credibility left that went when she disowned the contents of her own court statement, I looked over towards Laura Cox at that point and saw she had her head in both hands. I then looked over towards Des Kelly who looked back at me, he was a clammy

sickly grey, beads of sweat sat on his forehead. I hoped he could read what was in my eyes and my thoughts, "This is what you defended, this is what you let near the defenceless again and again, you deserve Maria Keenahan."When Ian Scott finished his cross examination of Maria Keenahan the Tribunal adjourned for a short break we all walked back to the waiting room, as soon as the door closed behind us Ian Scott turned to me and said "She was that bad and you were right, it's just so hard to believe that BUPA could spend five minutes with her and fail to see what she is" I said they know what she is, they have always known, they just did not want anyone else to know.

I had realised by that point that there were worse abusers than even Maria, as evil as she was. I knew those that could have stopped her abusing were the worst abusers of all. The more power to stop the abuse then the more guilt for not doing so. The first of these abusers to take the stand was Carole Jones who read both versions of her statements and was then cross examined. (Source, Barristers records)

"Mrs Jones, did you at any time care for residents with dementia prior to working at Isard House?"

"No"

"So in fact Eileen Chubb had more experience then you in dementia care?"

"Yes"

"Lets look at your statement paragraphs 31 to 33, you state here that, on March 31st, Eileen Chubb complained to me verbally that the medication trolley on unit three contained medication that was not prescribed and that medication was being withheld, I asked her not to repeat this to anyone and let me look into it, having informed no one of my intentions I visited unit three and carried out a full audit on unit three medication, is that your evidence to this Tribunal?"

"Yes as I said"

"Then you go on to state in paragraph 33 of your witness statement,
There were only some simple house keeping errors, when I informed Eileen Chubb of my findings and explained what I had found, she was most upset with me and I don't know why, I think she was disappointed with the fact that I had found very little of concern, certainly nothing to suggest any abuse of residents and that there was no need for me to take any action against Maria, that is your evidence?"

"Yes that is correct"

"But this is not true is it?"

"Yes it is"

Beyond The Facade

"A subsequent pharmacists report found plenty wrong and the medication sheets themselves show plenty was wrong?"

"I was told the drugs were not right and much like the inspectors I went and took a snapshot view of things.

"That's not what your witness statement says, I quote, I carried out a full audit on unit three medication, that's not a snapshot view is it?"

"It was a satisfactory inspection"

When Carole Jones had first entered the courtroom she was very confident and I had waited so long to hear her answer for what she had done. I suppose more than anything I wanted to know why, why would someone turn a blind eye to such terrible abuse. I watched her intently as the questions put to her slowly stripped away everything she had lied about.

"But you state there were only house keeping issues wrong"

"Yes"

"But it's simply not true?"

"At the time it's what I found"

"Lets look at the medication sheets of the resident

E.P (Edna), this sheet here, she is quite clearly not been given the right dose's is she?"

"I can not explain that"

"The dose prescribed on this sheet is much lower then what has been given, is it not?"

"No"

"Then what is stated as the dose that should be given?"

"Ten to twenty Mils"

"What has been given?"

"Thirty mils"

"Every single time"

"Yes"

"Three times a day"

"Yes"

"Please turn to the next sheet, this sheet is in fact a copy of the previous sheet, but a sticker has been placed over the existing G.P instructions?"

"Yes"

Beyond The Facade

"How did that happen?"

"I do not know"

"Then tell me what should have happened"

"The G.P should have signed to authorise the discontinued dosage and a new sticker placed in one of the empty spaces"

"But that is not what happened here is it?"

"No, the G.P must have forgotten to sign the sheet"

"So the G.P gave new instructions and forgot to sign the sheet and issued a new label, which then was accidentally stuck over the existing evidence of overdosing, is that what you are telling me?"

"That could have happened yes"

"Then explain the date on the label?"

We all held our breath and waited for Carole Jones to answer she opened her mouth several times but nothing came out, her eyes darted frantically around the room as if the answer lay there. I remembered Edna then as I had last seen her, the stench of neglect and her poisoned body racked with convulsions and her arm stretched out. I remembered Carole Jones telling me to trust her, she knew what was happening to Edna and the others she knew and did nothing. I did feel a bitter sweet satisfaction watching her now as she was faced with hard evidence from a barrister, a barrister that I had spent weeks training in medication procedures and now all that hard work was paying off.

"I said Explain to me Mrs Jones how an old label can cancel out existing G.P instructions?"

"I can not"

"Eileen Chubb reported this overdosing to you and then an out of date label appears covering up this overdosing?"

"I just can not explain that"

"But this was reported to you when Eileen Chubb told you the medication was not been correctly given"

"I did a snapshot inspection much the same as inspectors"

"When inspectors are investigating specific details of abuse, they do not do a snap shot inspection or they would not have uncovered all this?"

"I did an inspection"

"But you found nothing wrong did you?"

No response.

"I see, lets look at the earlier E.P (Edna) medication sheets which Eileen Chubb also reported to you, what about the overdosing here?"

"I rang the G.P to change the dose"

"Did you check on E.P?"

"I did not think it necessary to, the sheet was authorised by the G.P"

"Retrospectively of the overdosing?"

Again no response from Carole Jones her silence damned her more than any words could. By now she looked like a cornered animal and a film of sweat covered her face. Everything on the medication sheets had been reported to her and she did nothing about it. I remembered the last time I had gone to her for help and she told me that there was nothing wrong with the medication on unit three, I got up and walked away knowing I had to go outside the home for help because everything was wrong and anyone willing to look would see that.

"Answer the question Mrs Jones?"

"Yes"

"So a much earlier sheet shows serious

overdosing is taking place which Eileen Chubb reports to you and when she comes to you again months later with similar evidence of overdosing, you fail to see anything wrong?"

"I looked at the sheets"

"That is what worries me, these sheets show that not only were things wrong, they were very wrong indeed, weren't they?"

(No reply)

"Answer the question"

"I can not explain that"

"Lets look at Eileen Chubb's witness statement, paragraph 14 states,
in the summer of 98 when I moved back to unit three, I was appalled at the state of the medication, there was no records of medication in the trolley or what was being given to residents, there were controlled drugs which were not permitted, the drugs were out of date and in paragraph 31 the first overdosing, yes?"

"Yes"

"And in Eileen Chubb's statement, 38 and 45, I also reported misuse of medication yes?"

"Yes"

"Eileen Chubb was right to report these things to you?"

"I can not say"

"Mrs Jones looking at all the medication abuse here on these sheets, Eileen Chubb was right to report these things to you was she not?"

"Yes"

"But you took no action?"

"I did an inspection as I said"

"But you found nothing wrong did you?"

"No"

"Going back to your own witness statement, you say none of the other incidents of abuse was ever reported to you?"

"Yes"

"Lets look at the statement of Maria Keenahan, paragraph 60, the daughter of the resident A, removed A, from unit three, why was that Mrs Jones?"

"She was unhappy with her care"

"She sent you this letter dated 26th of March 1999?"

"Yes"

"She also sent copies of this letter to Des Kelly and Carole Newton?"

"Yes"

"This letter is listing among other things, lack of medical attention, loss of belongings, poor personal hygiene, her mothers hearing neglected, she goes on to state that she holds you personally responsible for her mothers Isolation and Deterioration and goes on to state, I would like to ask how you would feel enduring the same terrible pain and other symptoms, you have shown no consideration for the pain my mother was going through,
  This is not a letter about lack of care, it is yet another example of serious concerns being raised with you about unit three?"

"It was as I said"

  "Lets look again at Maria Keenahan's witness statement, paragraphs 94 to 96, she is stating here that, Big Maria came hot footing it down to tell me Linda Clark had reported me to Carole Jones for kicking the resident B.M,
Did Linda Clark report this to you?"

"No she did not"

"Linda Clark says she saw Maria Keenahan kicking the resident B.M hard and that she immediately reported this to you?"

"No she did not"

"Why is Maria Keenahan giving this version of events, is she lying?"

"I was not told"

"But you have such a high opinion of Maria and now you are saying she is a liar?"

"It was not reported to me"

"You say in your witness statement that Maria Keenahan is, kind generous and honest, but now you are saying she has not been honest about this?"

"I was not told"

We adjourned for lunch and once we were alone with the barrister, Ian Scott we all told him he was doing a great job, he said he was glad we approved with a smile.
We all went outside to get some air and we saw Carole Jones a little way off, she was talking to someone on her mobile and was crying, she turned away and went back inside when she saw

us and we all went over and sat on the wall pleased to be outside for a while but also wanting to get back for the cross examination to resume.

"Renee Warwick reported abuse to you as well?"

"No"

"Renee Warwick even demoted herself because of the abuse?"

"No I was going to demote anyway"

"That would amount to disciplinary action so you have file notes on this?"

"No"

"You were going to demote a member of staff but have not a single piece of documentary evidence to support such an action?"

"I have no notes as I said"

"It's simply not credible is it?"

"It's true"

"What would be the motive for the seven applicants making up the abuse?"

"I really can not say?"

Beyond The Facade

"Yet all seven applicants risked their jobs to report the abuse, why would they do that?"

There was a long pause and for some reason I noticed her shoes of all things and I thought her shoes probably cost more then the clothes all seven of us are wearing, God I thought I would rather be me with no knickers elastic then ever be her.

"I really do not know"

"What's your opinion of the Hair dresser who comes to the home?"

"She is good at her job"

"Would you say she was honest?"

"Yes I would"

"Lets look at the witness statement of the hairdresser she states that she saw a resident flinch from Sarah Conway, then realised that Sarah Conway was flicking food at the resident R.S, who asked her to stop, she goes on to state, Sarah had a funny way of caring for residents and had a big attitude problem. Yet Mrs Jones you have a very high opinion of Sarah Conway as well, do you believe she abused residents?"

"She may have been a little exuberant at times"

"Exuberant?"

"Yes"

"Looking at the hairdresser's statement, is that your idea of exuberance?"

"No"

"You say in your witness statement that suspending Sarah Conway was the hardest thing you have ever had to witness?"

"Yes it was very upsetting"

I could think of many upsetting things but which was the most upsetting, it could have been Edna's poisoned body racked by convulsions, perhaps it was Jessie her gangrenous gaping wound and the look in her eyes, pain beyond comprehension, I wished we could have a break, the cross examination was no longer giving me any satisfaction. Carole Jones had been exposed by the barrister long ago, I did not want to look at her or hear about her great compassion for abusers when she had shown no mercy for their victims, she was making me feel physically sick.

"As a professional nurse you must have seen many upsetting things, yet you say the suspension of Sarah Conway was the worst?"

"It was very upsetting"

"But Sarah Conway was being suspended on the grounds she may have been implicated in the most serious abuse of vulnerable residents?"

"It was hard to watch"

"I put it to you Mrs Jones that you had a closed mind from the start about the abuse and that you showed your anger to those who had dared to go outside the home with the concerns they had already reported to you repeatedly?"

"No"

"You had to discredit them for the fact they had gone to Social Services because they told you first?"

"No, I was not told"

"You instigated the resentment and watched the harassment of the applicants that followed as a result?"

"No"

At the end of her cross examination Carole Jones left the court, her employment references from BUPA were considered good enough for her to obtain work in further care homes, she is believed to be living in the Market Drayton area of Shropshire and managing a elderly care home in the area, there is nothing on her record to affect her fitness to hold this position.

Carole Newton was the next BUPA witness to read both versions of her witness statement and be cross examined. We all watched her intently as she crossed the room and took her seat in the witness box, she was a tall angular woman in her fifties with a long thin rather cruel looking face, young Lizzie had called her moggedy but she always reminded me of the wicked queen in Snow White.

"Mrs Newton were you aware of the abuse on unit three?"

"I was not aware and I spoke to residents and staff"

"When did you first become aware there were problems at Isard House?"

"When I was telephoned by inspection"

"So you were told serious allegations of abuse had been made?"

"I was told sweets had been stolen and I wondered what all the fuss was about"

"What was all the fuss about, Mr Turner has given evidence to this Tribunal that serious allegations of abuse were made and that you were informed

of this?"

"No"

"What did you think of Maria Keenahan?"

"I thought she was softly spoken and a very kind person"

"So when you were informed of the allegations against her you were very surprised?"

"Yes I was very surprised"

"I put it to you Mrs Newton that you had a closed mind from the start about any possibility that abuse had taken place?"

"I knew Maria Keenahan very well, I had spent a lot of time at the home when there was no manager, in the evenings, Maria was very helpful I do not think she could be involved in abuse"

"Lee Elkins says in his witness statement that you took him into the telephone room and told him to remember when he was interviewed by Social services, that Maria Keenahan had done nothing wrong?"

"That's not true I just wanted to reassure him"

This was the women who I had gone to for help, the only person we had access to who was in a position to help us, it had taken so few questions to expose her, it was clear that we never stood a chance of getting any help. She had made up her mind from the first day that we were making too much fuss about the abuse. I remembered how bad it was to go to work, how the job I had once loved had become this nightmare so bad that when the alarm clock went off in the mornings the first thing I did was cry at the thought I would have to walk into that place. I remembered walking through the door and a crowd would gather spitting threats so bad that my whole body would flinch from the blows I expected to rain down at any moment and there in the distance stood Carole Newton watching and smiling her approval.

"You arranged for Maria Keenahan to be placed at Anne Sutherland care home?"

"After an internal investigation it was decided to place her there"

"I refer you to the witness statement of Dick Turner, were you aware he was opposed to this?"

"We had an internal investigation and decided it was suitable to place Maria Keenahan there"

"Maria Keenahan was stopped from working at Anne Sutherland care home around the August Bank holiday, were you aware of that?"

"Yes Mr Kelly had spoken to me about placing her

at Faircroft instead"

"So you went ahead and placed her at Faircroft?"

"Yes it was suitable"

"Were you aware the staff records at Faircroft had been tampered with?"

"A member of staff panicked"

"Why would they panic if it was all above board?"

"They just panicked that's all"

"Were you involved with tampering with the records to hide Maria Keenahan's presence in the home?"

"There was an internal investigation and we saw no reason to keep her suspended"

"Mr Turners evidence to this Tribunal states, the manager of Faircroft, Mrs Edmonds has breeched the, Registered Homes Act, there is also the issue of tampering with records which reflected on her fitness and also on the fitness of the operational manager, Carole Newton, it was purely by chance that we discovered that Maria Keenahan was working at Faircroft, placing Maria Keenahan there was in breech of statutory regulations"

"We saw no reason to keep her suspended"

"Lets look at the independent pharmacists report, page after page of serious failings, in retrospect do you agree there were serious failings in the administration of medication?"

"No, It was just sloppy practice"

"Lets look at your own monthly drug audit's on Isard house, this one dated March 23rd 99, prior to the abuse being reported to Social Services, it consists of half a page of bullet points which say nothing was found to be wrong, not even sloppy practice?"

"It's what I saw"

"So then BUPA find out that serious allegations of abuse have been made including medication abuse and they carry out their own internal investigation into this?"

"Yes that is correct"

"This is that internal investigation report here?"

"Yes"

"A BUPA medication audit which was carried out by Susan Greenwood, BUPA's Quality Assurance Manager, her report is dated May 1999 and this is her report?"

"Yes"

"This report also consists of half a page of bullet points that find nothing wrong, is that so?"

"Yes"

"Looking at your earlier half page report which was made prior to the abuse being reported to Social Services, and then looking at this Susan Greenwood report, can you tell me where they differ?"

"I can not see"

"Your report on the medication and this later report are identical in every way, in fact they could be the same report if it were not for the dates?"

"As I said it's what I found"

"Is it not strange that both these half page reports are identical?"

"I really can not say"

"Was this internal BUPA medication audit that found nothing wrong used at Maria Keenahan's disciplinary interview?"

"Yes"

"The decision it was suitable to return Maria

Keenahan to work at firstly Anne Sutherland house and then at Faircroft two days later, was that based on this internal drug audit?"

"There was an investigation as I said"

"This investigation is this half page report is it not?"

"Yes"

"So you found nothing wrong before the abuse was reported to Social Services and after BUPA become aware of the allegations they come up with an identical report?"

"Yes"

"Just so I understand you correctly, six items are in order before the company is aware of the allegations and an identical six items are in order afterwards?"

"Yes"

"Pages and pages were wrong according to the independent Pharmacist report that was commissioned by Social Services?"

"We had our own internal investigation as I said"

Everything those residents had suffered was irrelevant as far as BUPA were concerned the only thing they ever cared about was that it be kept quite, the drug abuse alone was there for anyone willing to look, I could not help feeling angry that all that suffering was of no concern to them at all, even if they had publicly denied it and kept Little Maria from hurting anyone else that would have been at least something that I could understand, but knowing what this women was capable of they let her have access to yet more defenceless elderly people and all because protecting their reputation was the only thing they cared about. If we had not got those medical records out of the home that night they would have been destroyed and the truth buried. God they made me feel sick when I thought of Edna and the others, I remembered how Kitty screamed in pain after Maria stopped giving her painkillers.

"After the allegations were made you were asked by Carole Jones to speak with Eileen Chubb?"

"Yes I rang Eileen Chubb but she hung up so I went to speak to her at the home next day"

"Eileen Chubb says you were harassing her and following her around the unit?"

"No I just wanted to speak to her"

"Did you know she was one of the Whistle-blowers?"

"I suspected this, I told Des Kelly I thought she

was"

"So you attended a meeting later on that same day with Eileen Chubb, Dick Turner and Monica Handscomb?"

"Yes it was very strange, Eileen Chubb walked into the room and said I was harassing her"

"So she told you she felt harassed?"

"I thought she was distressed and should have gone home"

"Was the harassment investigated?"

"I rang the HR Department and arranged for a meeting to take place and for Eileen Chubb to have some time off"

"This meeting subsequently took place with Eileen Chubb, Linda Clark, yourself and Clair Porter from BUPA HR Department?"

"Yes"

"These are your own notes from that same meeting?"

"Yes they are"

"They state, Eileen Chubb said we are isolated and alone, feel threatened because we spoke out

and are working in appalling conditions?"

"They just wanted a platform to air their grievances"

"It appears to me that you would have suspended Eileen Chubb if she had not been one of the Whistle-blowers?"

"Yes prior to the meeting I did discuss suspending her with Mr Kelly"

"So even before you met with Eileen Chubb and heard her version of events, you had already decided she was the one at fault and required suspension?"

"As I have said I discussed it with Mr Kelly"

"So you just accepted Carole Jones version of events at face value and made up your mind it was Eileen Chubb who was at fault?"

"As I said"

"Why not suspend Carole Jones and Eileen Chubb and investigate both sides of the story?"

"It was Eileen Chubb who was the problem"

"I see, I have no further questions"

Carole Newton resigned from BUPA shortly after

the falsified records at Faircroft were discovered, she was last known to be working for a housing association.

Each of BUPA's witness's gave their evidence and were cross examined, as expected the abusers denied abusing, the harassers denied harassing and the managers denied everything. Finally there was only one witness left to take the stand, the most important witness of all Des Kelly.

Mr Kelly had been at the Tribunal every day of the hearing so we were used to seeing him, but it seemed strange to see him there in the witness box at last. Des Kelly was in his late forties with a bland face and receding hair line and had an unmistakable air of self importance about him, he was very fond of reciting his qualifications and achievements and referred to them throughout the pages of his written statements.

Mr Kelly read both versions of his witness statement and his cross examination began.

"Mr Kelly you state you were informed that sweets had been stolen from residents?"

"Yes"

"Can you please turn to the Social Services Inquiry report, pages and pages of the allegations that were made are listed here, residents pushed, kicked, spat at, residents shouted at, overdosed,

page after page of the most horrific abuse, but like Carole Newton you were only informed sweets were stolen?"

"Yes as I said"

"It's quite clear that as far as you were concerned any abuse reported was not true and that was the position you took from the outset?"

"As I said"

"When this attitude is taken from the outset, when allegations of abuse are made, then it is hardly surprising that an identical approach is taken to allegations of harassment?"

"I was not informed of any harassment"

"You say you were not informed of the abuse either?"

"As I have said"

"When were you first aware that Social Services and the police were going to ascend on Isard House regarding these missing sweets?"

"I was informed by Carole Newton on April 20th 1999"

"Did you go to Isard House?"

"No not then, I visited later and spoke to staff informally, it was decided that Carole Newton should remain at Isard House"

"Did Carole Newton inform you of the meeting that took place with herself and Eileen Chubb and Clair Porter?"

"Yes she said it was very distressing and I asked her to provide me with a written file note"

"So you saw her notes of this meeting?"

"Yes"

"What did you make of them?"

"I thought Eileen Chubb seemed very distressed"

"What about the words, We feel Isolated and alone?"

"As I said I thought she was distressed"

"What about the words, We feel threatened because we spoke out?"

"As I said"

"What did you think they could have spoken out about that could result in them, working in the Appalling conditions mentioned here?"

"We suspected they may have been the whistle-blowers but there was nothing about harassment"

"It never occurred to you that Eileen Chubb might be asking for help?"

"No it did not seem that way to me"

"I see, the meeting of May 14th you were to meet with all seven applicants?"

"No only two, Eileen Chubb and Linda Clark"

"But you met with all seven?"

"Yes"

"Mr Turner of Social Services attended this meeting also?"

"Yes"

"Mr Turner has given evidence to this Tribunal that the applicants behaved very professionally at this meeting with you?"

"That is not my recollection, my recollection is that they were all talking at once"

"Did the applicants tell you they were being harassed?"

"No they did not, I only recall Eileen Chubb saying

she had been pushed in the back"

"Why would Eileen Chubb tell that she had been hit with a chair, if the harassment was not being discussed?"

"They were all talking at once as I said"

I found the hardest part sitting there and not being able to say anything, I thought it would be clear you are asking for help if you tell someone you are working in appalling conditions and feel threatened for speaking out. I know we did everything we could to get help but it was obvious that we were seen as the problem for reporting the abuse in the first place.

"As such an experienced manager you must have come across abuse before?"

"Yes I have"

"You must have then been aware that harassment of Whistle-blowers is a very common problem in such situations?"

"Yes I am aware that can happen"

"But you did not think it could be happening in this case?"

"I had not seen any indication of this, one might feel isolated but I do not think seven could"

"But harassment of Whistle-blowers is a very real danger you just agreed?"

"Yes I was aware"

"I need you to be very clear on this point, Social Services would not be responsible for investigating harassment would they"

"No it would not be their responsibility"

"So if you received complaints of harassment it is you who should have investigated?"

"That is correct"

"Now I need you to be quite clear on this point also, at any time has there ever been an investigation into the harassment the applicants reported?"

"There has been no investigation no"

"At any time?"

"No, Never"

"Did you never consider taking any action on the harassment?"

"I had no opportunity to, I thought we should see the seven staff separately"

"Why separately?"

"Because of my experience of them as a group"

"Mr Turner was at this meeting and he made notes, his evidence to this Tribunal is clear and I quote from his witness statement,
On May 5th Eileen Chubb telephoned me for assistance because she was being chased around Isard House by Carole Newton, the BUPA operational manager and she had locked herself in a residents bedroom to get away from her, as this breakdown in the relationship between manager and staff member was affecting the running of the home, Monica Handscomb and I attended Isard House immediately. Eileen Chubb had contacted us in order to try and keep the peace and avoid too much disruption. An interview took place between Eileen Chubb and Carole Newton in the conference room, myself and Monica Handscomb were Present"

"The meeting was for Carole Newton to establish what the problem had been and it appeared she saw Eileen Chubb as the ring leader, Eileen Chubb was too distraught to go on working, I felt we were mediating in an internal employer/employee situation which could not be resolved easily and was not our role. Carole Newton asked why Eileen Chubb had gone to Social Services when there was a BUPA help-line for carers, Monica Handscomb pointed out that

there was no such help-line at the time and when they had brought concerns to the management nothing had happened. Eileen Chubb indicated to Monica Handscomb that she could not go on working under the circumstances and Monica told Carole Newton she agreed with this. Mr Kelly was BUPA's Director, Carole Newton was the area manager, Mr Kelly was therefore her line manager. I suggested to him he should attend a meeting with the Whistle-blowers as a way of reducing their tension and distress. I told him that I believed the staff group had come to us in good faith, I was concerned if this disruption was going to continue at Isard House it would affect the residents.

I arranged for the meeting to take place on May 14th, the meeting was attended by all seven Whistle-blowers, Mr Kelly and myself, Monica Handscomb joined us later, it was a very constructive meeting in the sense the Whistle-blowers were reasonably calm and very professional"

"My recollection is people were crying"

"Do go on Mr Kelly?"

"They did a presentation and then it developed into everyone talking at once"

"You took notes?"

"No"

"Very odd"

"Yes I suppose, I only thought two were coming"

"But even if you thought only two were coming you would have still gone prepared?"

"I felt I was set up the way it was done, I thought I was only meeting with two staff not seven with a presentation, I was listening but I took no notes, that is because of the way it was done"

"Look again at Dick Turners statement, The meeting was very constructive, is what he is saying?"

"It is not what I recall, I recall a lot of emotion"

"Why should there not be some emotion in the circumstances?"

"They were all talking at once"

"Not according to Dick Turner?"

"That is what I recollect"

Mr Kelly seemed very relieved when we adjourned for lunch, we all told Ian Scott he was doing great, and I asked would it have been our word against his if Social Services had not been present at that meeting with Des Kelly, Ian said, "yes but they were present and are independent witness's and have no motive to lie, Mr Kelly on the other hand has every reason to lie." The cross examination continued after lunch.

"When Eileen Chubb told you she had been hit in the back with a chair, is that not a serious assault on a member of staff?"

"Yes but she said it during other things, it got missed in the meeting"

"Did you follow it up at any later time?"

"No as I said it got missed"

"You recalled it clearly enough to put it in your witness statement?"

"As I said"

"Did Eileen Chubb mention being hit during other examples of harassment?"

"No, that was the only thing mentioned"

"It seems an odd thing to come out with?"

I remembered the force of that chair smashing into my back, I only got through the rest of that shift because I was in some kind of shock and it was only when I got home that night that the full impact hit me, everything we had gone through and then we get a meeting with Mr Kelly and I am supposed to have forgotten to tell him about the harassment, what was I supposed to have talked about the weather? Oh and by the way Mr Kelly someone smashed a chair into my back. I did feel angry having to sit and listen to this man lying through his teeth not only because he could have helped us but chose not to, but because he could have helped the residents.

"They were all talking at once"

"Were you aware that the other staff in the home were angry?"

"I spoke to the staff on May 19th, there seemed to be, and also some fear over loosing their jobs"

"Did the seven staff tell you they were sick when you met with them?"

"I must have known they were sick but I can not recollect how I knew"

"Did you not think it was odd all seven staff off sick at once?"

"Yes it was unusual"

"Did you not try to find out why they were all sick?"

"I thought the meeting was about the abuse"

"Let us look at Dick Turners witness statement again, he states that,
On May 24th I arranged for the Whistle-blowers to have counselling through a voluntary organisation, I was conscious that my lines of responsibility were becoming blurred, I felt sorry for the Whistle-blowers, who had come to us in good faith, wanting to help them, but at the same time I did not want their concerns treated as gossip. There was a need to ensure their emotional needs were receiving help from external sources and that their health was protected.
Was it Mr Turner's responsibility to safeguard their health?"

"No it would not be his role, no"

"Mr Turner could see they were in need of help, could you not see the same?"

"I do not recall how I knew they were sick as I said"

"The seven gave you a chart on May 14th, which you took away with you, what was that about?"

"I did take the chart away, I do not recall what it was about, something to do with abusers who were problem staff"

"You never looked at this chart even when you recovered it, to submit in evidence?"

"No as I said"

"This chart clearly identifies two separate staff groups, the abusers and then the problem staff and how they were inter-related?"

"It was my recollection that the chart was about abusers"

"Why would the seven go to all the trouble of making this chart for you?"

"I really could not say"

"Has this chart at any time since being examined by yourselves with a view to investigating the harassment?"

"There has been no investigation, no"

"I see, lets look at the Council minutes for May 13th 1999, they say on 119, Des Kelly said it's complicated because of the two Maria's, Carole Jones response was indeed inadequate, is that correct?"

"I could not say for certain"

"What about the top of page 4, Des Kelly says we can all make mistakes, Maria was not telling the truth, is that correct?"

"It sounds like something I may have said"

"It then continues, Des Kelly said there are two groups of staff and I can not satisfy both, is that correct?"

"I did not know there were two groups of staff, I do not know how I could have said that"

"The Bromley Council Clerk, who recorded these minutes has no reason to make things up, do you agree?"

"Yes, but I do not know how I could have said that"

"Maybe the file notes you asked Carole Newton to provide you with would explain how you knew that there were two groups of staff, the ones who, Felt threatened for speaking out and who were working in, appalling Conditions, and the other group of staff who were causing those conditions?"

"No"

"Carole Newton gave you these files notes, that is what you have stated in your witness statement?"

"Yes I think she did give them"

"You can not explain how you could have said on May 13th that you knew about the two staff groups?"

"No I do not know how I could have known that"

"But you do know with certainty that Carole Newton's notes could not be the explanation?"

"I can only say what I have said already"

*"I see. Lets turn over the page and return to the minutes taken by the Council Clerk, which state, Des Kelly said as soon as the legal team come into it, it will not matter what has gone on here, they will go all defensive,
is that correct?"*

"It's true in parts, the main recommendation in the draft report was the home should be de-registered and the legal team would have become involved"

"The home should be closed was the main recommendation in the draft report?"

"Yes"

"Lets look at the letter sent to the applicants solicitors in response to their letter to Sir Brian Nickolson, what is clearly being said here in this letter from your legal department that, all the applicants made references to being harassed when they met with Des Kelly on May 14th, where did your legal department get that information from?"

"I must have gave them a report of the meeting"

"So they relied on your report of this meeting in order to write this response to the applicant's solicitors?"

"Yes"

"But they are saying here that all seven applicants made reference to being harassed?"

"I can not explain that, I only recollect E. Chubb saying she was pushed, I can not understand that"

"You can give no possible explanation as to why your own legal Department would say that?"

"No I can not explain that"

"Going back to the Bromley Council Clerks minutes, there is a reference there about you meeting with all seven staff?"

"Well I have my doubts about that"

"But you agreed earlier that the clerk would have no reason to make things up?"

"Yes but I can not have said that"

"Returning to your original witness statement, you say the management approach was to support Carole Jones?"

"Yes"

"I believe you sat through Mrs Jones cross examination?"

"Yes"

"When you took the decision to support Carole Jones were you aware she had been accused of failing to act on abuse that was reported to her?"

"I must have been at some stage yes"

"Did it ever occur to you that Carole Jones may feel anger towards those who had accused her of such serious failings?"

"I do not recollect exactly"

God I thought this man has got a worse memory than most of the residents in Isard House and yet he remembers enough to deny everything. Carole Jones was in a position of power and she used that position to make our lives hell.

"Carole Jones says in her statement that, Chocolates were bought for all the staff and Des Kelly visited later that day to offer his support, This is the same day the applicants were forced out of the building?"

"I believe it was their first day of sickness yes"

"The day the applicants went sick was the day staff were bought chocolates?"

"Yes"

"The day the applicants went sick was the day you visited?"

"I had visited previously as well"

"But bypassed unit two completely on that first visit?"

"I do not recollect exactly who was spoken to now"

"Further down that page it says, Maria Green said if the applicants go back to work the staff will rebel, is that a recognition the applicants could not return to work?"

"I was alive to the fact they could be placed in other care homes when they returned from sick leave yes?"

"Why should the seven be moved to other care homes, they had done nothing wrong?"

"I do not recollect the exact circumstances now"

"Those who were accused of abuse were suspended on full pay whilst the applicants were only paid sick pay?"

"Yes we fulfilled our contractual obligations and they would not meet with us"

"The applicants were always willing to meet as a group, why would your H.R Department not meet with them as a group?"

"I had formed the view it would not be suitable"

"Did you ever think of reviewing that decision?"

"It was my experience of them as a group"

"Your experience of them as a group is very different to Mr Turners who attended the meeting as an independent observer and who took notes?"

"I can only say it was not my experience of them"

"Yet you are totally contradicted by Mr Turner's evidence?"

"I do not know why they were so suspicious of meeting one to one"

"The applicants were always willing to meet as a group but as a result of your recommendations H.R refused to meet with them?"

"As I already said"

"At any time from receiving the final inquiry report did you make any formal complaints about Mr

Turner's investigation?"

"I have this letter"

"No I mean in the eighteen months prior to you having sight of Mr Turner's statement to this Tribunal?"

"No"

We adjourned until the next day and we all went home confident that Mr Kelly looked like the liar he was, hard evidence contradicted him at every turn. I looked forward to the next day and had prepared my usual list of questions for the barrister to ask, I really wanted to know why BUPA allowed little Maria to work in their homes, why known abusers were promoted and protected by them when they would not lift a finger to help us.

"Let's turn to Mr Turners letters to you regarding the re-deployment of Maria Keenahan, I quote "Maria Keenahan should remain suspended" Another letter here he states "Keep Maria Keenahan suspended our concerns are extensive, you will have all the information, she was involved in abuse, her care practices are subject, I pass this matter to our solicitors"

"He is saying that he knew nothing about Faircroft?"

"I do not think there is much difference between

Mr Turners View and mine, I accept it was not suitable, I accept the company can be criticised for not telling Social Services, but not for placing Maria Keenahan in another home, we should have told them"

"This has nothing to do with not telling them, this is about ignoring Social Services when they clearly told you not to re-employ Maria Keenahan, it is quite clearly stated here?"

"He is only saying that now"

"Lets read again Mr Turners evidence to this Tribunal on the matter, Mr Turner states, On the 27th of August 1999 I received information via one of the managers of another care home in the BUPA group, who reported to Monica Handscomb that Maria Keenahan was to be re-employed at Anne Sutthererland House, in a similar capacity to that she held at Isard house. It was around the same date I also received a call from Eileen Chubb stating Maria Keenahan was due to be re-employed at Anne Sutherland House as a team leader on a unit for the elderly mentally infirm, (EMI) at the time Maria Keenahan was on police bail for theft whilst police made further inquiries"

"We managed to ascertain that Maria Keenahan was due to start work on Tuesday 31st of August 1999, after the bank holiday Monday.
Over Saturday 28th and Sunday 29th of August, I contacted Des Kelly at his home and said that the

re-deployment of Maria Keenahan at Anne Sutherland was unacceptable to us, especially as she was firstly on bail for theft and secondly in our view she was implicated in both abuse and neglectful behaviour, either by both herself and members of her team on the unit she was managing, Mr Kelly ultimately agreed to prevent her commencing employment at Anne Sutherland house, I phoned Anne Sutherland house to confirm this was the case.

On the 1ˢᵗ of December 1999, E. Chubb and K. Hook came to the civic centre, with information that Maria Keenahan was working at Faircroft"

"Faircroft operated under a separate company in the BUPA group and was for entirely mentally infirm (EMI) residents, I rang and asked to speak to Mrs Lydia Edmonds the manager, I asked her if she had a Maria Keenahan working there which she denied, I was not satisfied with her reply so I visited the home that evening to coincide with the changeover of staff for night shift. Monica Handscomb and myself looked at the records from which it appears the rotas had been altered and the name, Maria tipexed out on at least one of those we seen. These rotas were hanging in the office upstairs, further were held in the managers office in the basement which we did not have access to that evening.

We returned at eight thirty next morning and waited for the manager to arrive at nine fifteen, we interviewed her and she finally agreed that Maria Keenahan had worked there since September

1999, Mrs Edmonds said she knew Maria Keenahan was on bail for theft, she was unaware of the allegations of verbal and physical abuse made against her, Maria Keenahan herself had told her about these weeks later, the manager was under the impression that Maria Keenahan had been discriminated against for race reasons and she felt sympathy towards her.

Carole Newton had brought Maria Keenahan to Faircroft when the manager was off duty, we subsequently ascertained this had occurred on the 31st of August 99, immediately after we prevented her from working at Anne Sutherland house, Mrs Edmonds had not raised the issue, it was her view there was not a shred of evidence to back up the allegations.

I wrote to Peter Ludford the BUPA operational director he did not reply, I drew attention to the fact that Maria Keenahan's was on bail and this information was included in detail in my letter of December 21st 99.

I now understand that from June 2000 Maria Keenahan was re-suspended. And is no longer working at Faircroft, my letters were passed to Mr Kelly for a reply without any acknowledgement from Mr Ludford.

Mr Turner is quite clearly shocked to Find Maria Keenahan at Faircroft?"

"I accept there is a difference of opinion between Mr Turner and myself, but he escalates the fact she should not work with the elderly, it was only in December that we were told of his feelings

regarding Maria Keenahan, it was up to us we were her employers"

"So you agreed with Mr Turner in August that she should not start work at Anne Sutherland house and the next day you send her to Faircroft knowing Mr Turner thought her a danger?"

"Faircroft is not a contracted out home"

"That has nothing to do with it, abuse can happen in any home?"

"I saw no evidence to keep her suspended"

Des Kelly looked a sickly grey colour which was hardly surprising as he knew what was coming next, he had sat through all the cross examinations and knew his every attempt to cover-up the abuse had failed, against the odds we had not only got the evidence out of the home but had made it to a court hearing where it could all be exposed publicly. Mr Kelly looked like a man who had dug himself a hole and now faced with the truth he could hold his hands up and admit he was wrong or he could carry on digging, it was obvious he had decided on the latter.

"Let's examine the evidence you did have at the time, are you familiar with medication records?"

"Our Quality Assurance Department deals with that"

"Were you not present through out Mrs Newton's cross examination?"

"Yes"

"So you are aware of the medication audit Mrs Newton carried out prior to the allegations of abuse, lets turn to that now, this is it?"

"Yes"

"Over the page this is the internal investigation that you carried out?"

"Yes"

"Both these audit's consist of six bullet points on half a page which conclude nothing is wrong?"

"Yes"

"You have seen the comprehensive report by the independent pharmacist?"

"Yes"

"Which of these two audit's did you use at Maria Keenahan's Disciplinary hearing?"

"We used our internal audit"

"The independent pharmacists audit bears no

resemblance in volume or content to your six bullet point audit?"

"We relied on our own audit, the independent pharmacist never said the abuse was deliberate"

"It was not the pharmacists remit to investigate the intent but only to account for the drugs that came in, went out and were given?"

"I relied on our report"

"Lets look at the notes of your disciplinary hearing with Maria Keenahan, the vast amount of questions here seem to be about Eileen Chubb?"

"Yes"

"It looks to me as if you were you investigating Eileen Chubb and not Maria Keenahan at all?"

"Her medication practices were put to her"

"So if we turn over the pages on Eileen Chubb, we at last come to some of the questions put to her, she is not pressed at all on the medication abuse?"

"We found no evidence of that"

"Not in your investigation audit but you could have used both audit's?"

"As I said we decided to use our own audit"

"The one that found nothing wrong, I see. Let's return to Maria Keenahan being placed at Anne Sutherland house, why was that done?"

"It was decided it was suitable to return her to work"

"Lets look at this letter dated September 6th 1999, it's from Bromley Social Services to yourselves it states, I stopped Maria Keenahan from working at Anne Sutherland house, the return of Maria Keenahan to any care home will become a matter for our legal department, you knew this and yet still re-employed this women at Faircroft?"

"The responsibilities we had with contracted out homes did not apply to Faircroft, the inquiry report said Maria Keenahan should not work with E.M.I residents, this letter implies other then this"

"What category of residents are cared for at Faircroft Mr Kelly?"

"As I said Faircroft is not a contracted out home"

"Please answer the question Mr Kelly, what category of residents are cared for at Faircroft?"

"E.M.I"

The most defenceless residents are E.M.I, like

Jessie they are often unable to tell anyone what's happening to them and that's why they are often the preferred victims of power abusers like Maria, all that stood between Maria and the most defenceless was this man Mr Kelly, he knew what Maria was capable of and let her near more defenceless people, but the worse thing was his motive for doing so, his actions were not the result of some kind of oversight or misunderstanding but a deliberate cover-up. BUPA always knew we were telling the truth but to acknowledge Maria was a abuser would have been to publicly acknowledge the abuse and that would damage their reputation, so more defenceless people were left at Maria's mercy and every time I thought of Maria I saw her cold twisted face full of anticipation for the torture she was about to inflict and I wondered why someone could allow that for the sake of their reputation, I wondered what reputation was worth that and I knew this company was rotten to the core.

"Let us return to the insufficient evidence you had to keep Maria Keenahan suspended, You used your own internal drugs audit to question Maria Keenahan?"

"Yes"

"You declined to use the damming independent pharmacist's audit?"

"As I said, we used our own internal audit"

"You decided that there was insufficient evidence to keep Maria Keenahan suspended and intend to return her to work at Anne Sutherland house?"

"As I said she gave nothing in her responses to cause concern"

"That is hardly surprising when you consider what was put to her?"

"I did ask her if she had anything to say"

"Then against all the odds at the end of this disciplinary meeting Maria Keenahan says to you, that she judged what dosage to give to E.P and that she told the management what she was doing, she tells you this according to your own notes?"

"Yes it was said"

"Just so I understand you correctly, you ask Maria Keenahan if she wants to say anything and she tells you she is prescribing drugs with the managements knowledge and you do not pursue this at all?"

"We did not have the understanding of the medication records then that we now have"

"Even when you were in possession of Eileen Chubb's witness statement which shows her

understanding of the medication records, even then you placed Maria Keenahan in another care home?"

"As I have already said. We had another investigation too"

"That was much later and still found nothing of concern?"

"That is correct"

"At no time were the allegations of harassment ever investigated?"

"No"

"You were having no truck with those allegations either were you?"

"As I said I was not told about the harassment"

"You were somehow not informed of the abuse either, stolen sweets was it not?"

"That's what I was told"

"I see, I have no further questions for this witness"

Questions from the bench. (Mrs Greenman)

"The meeting of May 14th, Mr Kelly did you ask the applicants why they were sick?"

"I thought I was only to meet with two because of the nature of the meeting I felt I could not pursue why they were sick"

"But all seven staff sick and you did not ask why?"

"I did not think it appropriate to ask them"

"That's what worries me, you never wrote to them after the meeting?"

"No"

"At no time"

"No, I contacted HR"

"But it's you that met with them is it not usual that it should have been you that wrote to them?"

"I felt HR should deal with it"

Question from the bench (Mr Zuke)

"Could you look at b.4 Mr Kelly, these are notes of an interview with yourself and Carole Jones, you ask her if there is evidence of a member of staff being assaulted, is that an accurate note?"

"Yes it is"

Des Kelly later resigned from BUPA and is

currently the director of The National Care Forum, which represents the interests of the care industry at Government level.
(In 2007 Des kelly was awarded the OBE for services to the care industry and in December 2007 he was voted " Care personality of the year")

So at last all the evidence was heard, I think we all felt huge relief at that but also we felt exhausted, I did not know how we managed to make it through it had been so hard. We were just so happy to have got this far that it did not seem that bad when the case had to be adjourned yet again due to there being no time left for the barristers closing arguments or written submissions. What mattered most was that all the evidence had been heard and in spite of every starve out tactic and obstacle, we had made it through against all the odds. We all felt really confident and never doubted for a moment that we had won, the solicitor, Sarah Culshaw and barrister, Ian Scott, were equally confident, how could we not be when we had all the evidence and all BUPA had was denial every step of the way.

So the case was adjourned until June 4th 2001 which was the earliest date the Tribunal could fit us in, the last thing Ian Scott told us before we all went home was, "You are the perfect Whistle-blowers, you have done the right thing and the law will protect you." We were never to see him again as we did not return to the Tribunal. Now that all the evidence had been heard, the solicitor Sarah

Culshaw agreed when I asked if I could now take this evidence to the police again. It seemed clear there were sufficient grounds to re-open the case. I had never understood why Maria Keenahan had only been questioned about theft when there was all the evidence on the medication abuse. I had started to think that perhaps the police had not understood the significance of the medical records and if they had some help to understand them then they would act. So I spent days indexing all the evidence into three large ring binders, with a separate section for each victim, which contained that persons medication records, a full typed step by step guide to each separate medication sheet, which explained in simple terms how the drugs were illegally stockpiled and how lethal doses had been administered. I also researched every single drug and included copies of all the relevant pages from the medical text books. I had spent months training the barrister on how to understand drug sheets and that experience served me well now. I took these three folders, which contained well over a thousand pages of hard factual evidence, along with the contact details of seven witness's willing to testify in court to Bromley Police station. I kept ringing the Police at regular intervals only to be told there was no one on duty involved with the case that I could speak to. I was informed quite some time later that the C.P.S had decided there was insufficient evidence to bring a case, despite the fact that none of the witnesses were ever interviewed. I was stunned to hear this as I knew the evidence was there and I could not understand this at all, I took it further but to no avail. The hardest part of this was that it resulted in BUPA continually issuing public statements saying the Police had investigated and found nothing wrong. In effect the Police gave BUPA a shield to hide behind.

I never doubted that the law would be on the side of right and truth, it was the summer of 2001 and we all received copies of our barrister's submissions and waited for the Tribunal verdict.

Extracts from the written submissions of, Ian Scott. (Please see index)

While we waited for the Tribunal verdict, we were contacted by the daughter of Audrey Ford, who had been one of our residents on unit two, Audrey's daughter, Dylas said her mother had been admitted to hospital suffering from the side effects of Anti Psychotic drugs. Dylas asked if we would come and visit her mother at Orpington hospital, she tried to prepare us and told us before we went in, "Do not expect to see the plump happy women you knew as Audrey, she is now less then seven stone and a drugged wreck" But nothing could have prepared us for the women we saw lying in that hospital bed, we all cried when we saw her, she was a bag of bones wearing a nightdress that had once fitted her stocky frame but which now hung in huge folds which only emphasised the shrunken women it enveloped like a shroud. I told Audrey I was sorry, so sorry that we had not done enough to protect her, as I sat by her bed and watched her sleep, I thought the Tribunal verdict will come any day now and BUPA will receive some measure of justice for what they have done, it was July 2001.

The end we had all longed for was not to be, in fact the real fight was only just beginning, on Saturday July 21st 2001, The Employment Tribunal verdict arrived in the post.
I sat down to read it and as I turned the pages I remembered another Saturday, nearly two and a half years earlier, when I had sat writing a statement about abuse, I had cried then as well but this was something much worse, after everything we had gone through. I could hardly breathe as I read the words, the words that I had waited so long to hear. I sat in stunned silence while Steve read the verdict, I hoped it was all a huge mistake and that Steve would tell me anytime now that it was alright really, when he finally finished reading he looked up and said. "This has got to be deliberate, no one could make that many mistakes". It was only then that the full impact slammed into me. "Who will believe us they will say, a judge said it so it must be true. "I said and then we both just sat there in stunned silence for a long time, staring at the verdict as if it were all part of a bad dream and we would wake up and laugh about it soon. Steve was the first to break the long silence, "If you do not fight this you will

damn all those who come after".

I suppose life always comes down to two choices in the end, you can sit down and cry or stand up and fight and I did sit down and cry that Saturday, but not for long. The others rang me throughout the morning, I heard the same hopeless despair in their voices, that I had felt just a short while earlier and I tried to give what comfort I could, we all decided to fight on after all we had nothing to lose.

I set the alarm clock that night for six am on Sunday morning, I had already been typing a couple of hours when I heard it go off. We were all going to formally respond to the verdict in writing and I felt so overwhelmed by the sheer volume of evidence that was missing that I never thought I would be able to list it all, I was still typing at ten o'clock that night.

What we all found the hardest thing to bear was the verdicts attacks on the residents, who could no more defend themselves from these criticisms than they could defend themselves from the abuse, the verdict did one of two things when it came to the abuse, firstly it justified and excused it to such an extent that it fabricated evidence to do so, for example when the Tribunal had to choose between two conflicting accounts of an incident such as,
A. Linda Clark said she saw Maria Keenahan kick a resident.
or

B. Maria Keenahan totally denies she kicked the resident.

The Tribunal has to choose between A or B but instead it ignores both versions of the event and fabricates evidence to conclude the following.

"The resident kicked Maria Keenahan who then kicked her back but with only a slight degree of force"

In doing this the Tribunal gave Maria Keenahan a reason a kick a defenceless old women by blaming the victim for instigating the assault. Nearly all of the abuse that was included in the verdict was dealt with in the same way.

The second thing the verdict did was to suppress any evidence that could not easily be justified and excused and so conflicted with their conclusions. Our whole case for reasonable belief was demonstrated by using particular examples, in the case of the medication abuse, the records belonging to Edna were used, as they clearly showed the deliberate overdosing that BUPA were aware of and tried to cover up. So how did the Tribunal deal with all of the evidence relating to Edna? It could not excuse it, so it made not one single reference to the fact that it ever existed in the first place.

Des Kelly could not be considered a credible witness whilst the evidence of Edna's abuse existed, so the Tribunal suppressed it, and then went on to conclude the following,

Beyond The Facade

The Tribunal found Mr Kelly to be a credible witness, for the following reasons

The verdict concludes Mr Kelly met with the applicants on May 14th and they did not tell him about any harassment.

The verdict concludes Mr Kelly immediately arranged counselling for the applicants after his meeting with them.

The verdict concludes that the BUPA internal drug audit and the independents pharmacists written reports agreed that nothing of concern was found.

The verdict concludes that we should have given more thought to our own positions before we went and reported the abuse.

The verdict concludes Mr Kelly did not place Maria Keenahan in the care home Faircroft in August.

Carole Newton is mentioned once, but neither her own notes nor her evidence are referred to at all, the following words are all that is mentioned "Carole Newton only wanted to speak to Eileen Chubb."

All of the independent Witness statements are suppressed as is all the evidence of Dick Turner including the findings of his inquiry report. The Tribunal made no mention of the fact that I

reported the harassment to Carole Newton and H.R, in fact there was no mention of anything that made BUPA look bad, in all over one hundred separate pieces of independent documentary evidence was suppressed, each piece contradicted the Tribunals conclusions in full.
I thought I would never get to the end of the list and I felt huge relief when I finally finished typing nearly fourteen hours later.

The Phone started ringing at nine o'clock that Monday morning. I knew it would be the solicitor, Sarah Culshaw even before I heard her voice asking me if I got the verdict in the post. I told her I was posting a formal written response and she would have it by the next day and that the verdict was disputed in full. There was a long silence and then she said in a very shaky voice that I could not do that as a remedial hearing date was set and the Tribunal would be awarding us money, she went on to say how BUPA did not want this to happen and would pay me anything I wanted to settle now. She paused for a split second before she added in a casual voice, that she would be paid seventy thousands pounds by BUPA towards her own costs on the condition that she advised us to settle.
"So that's how it works, no win, no fee, whose interests are being served yours or ours" I said. She started beseeching me and said "The others will settle if you do and Eileen you can buy new clothes and have a nice holiday." I asked her where I could possibly go to on holiday that did not

have mirrors so I could avoid looking into my own eyes." I could feel the anger rising and I reminded her we had never gone into court for money, but for justice. "Do you think I went through all this for that Tribunal to say the abuse was alright and we should have considered our jobs before we reported it?" I shouted.

I could hear the anger in her voice, the desperation for her promised seventy thousand pounds, but only if she sold us out. She shouted at me angrily, "You must have a price everyone has a price", and suddenly I was back in Isard House, the smell of torture in my nostril's and Edna's hand reaching out, and in a deadly calm voice I said, "This is my final answer, you can tell BUPA I have no price, they do not have enough money to keep me quite and you are sacked" I put the phone down and I realised I had learned something about myself. Most people will never be asked what their price is but it is only then that you realise there are some things beyond price, BUPA have still to learn that.

I had no idea where we were going to get help from and someone suggested that I try contacting a Charity called, Public Concern at Work, who had written the Public Interest Disclosure Act. So I wrote a long letter to them explaining our situation and enclosing a copy of the verdict and my response, which listed all we disputed. I said that I would telephone once they had some time to read the documents and I rang them a short while later.

I spoke to a man called Guy Dehn, who was immediately hostile and so defensive about his law. "You should have settled with BUPA, why did you go to court with this law?" he shouted at me angrily. I said it was obvious he could not help and as soon as I put the phone down. I thought there is something really wrong with that law, that man is only interested in protecting his reputation, not Whistle-blowers. "That Guy Dehn wouldn't know what harassment was if it came up and bit him on the arse, honestly these people." I was pacing up and down in a rage, God I was so different it was like my whole personality had changed. Steve stood staring at me in disbelief, I was the last person to see how much I had changed but I knew right then I had crossed some kind of line and I was not a victim any more. I wrote a polite letter to Guy Dehn a few days later. I said that I hoped other Whistle-blowers who had the misfortune to need his help-line, received better treatment then I did. I told him that, his Public Interest Disclosure Act was not worth the paper it was written on and it was small wonder he did not want it used in court. He wrote back and denied he had said any of it and that he would be happy for any suggestions I had for improving the service his Charity offered. I replied and said I had taped him and as to improving his Charity, he could give his job to someone else. He wrote back and said it was illegal to tape people, "not if it's in the public interest it's not" I replied and that was the end of that. I never heard from him again but I have since learnt of other Whistle-blowers who have given up disheartened after speaking to Mr Dehn, which is hardly surprising.

I went to a book shop in Bromley and bought a reduced copy of, The Penguin Guide To The Law, which was only £3.99, God that has got to be the best £3.99 that I ever spent. Sarah Culshaw would not give us the evidence bundles and I tried to wheedle them out of the Clerk at Ashford and nearly got them too but for Mr Zuke getting wind of it.

Fortunately we had all taken a keen interest in the evidence and between all seven of us, we had copies of all the evidence and I had the bundle indexes. Everyone brought over their documents and put ten pounds in a kitty, which Steve and I used to photo copy everything and we spent nearly a week working until gone midnight assembling all the bundles from scratch, which was a huge task but we did it. We then received a hearing date from the Ashford Tribunal for what they called, the remedial hearing, which is when they award money to us based on the verdict. We had already informed the Tribunal that we disputed the verdict in full and would accept no compensation as we could never accept a verdict that excused abuse. So we were surprised they intended to hold such a hearing in the circumstances and wrote to them again informing them we were going to appeal and requested they suspend the hearing until the appeal, as they had done so readily for BUPA, when they had appealed. It seemed a fair request but it was refused. I met Heather Mills, from Private Eye for the first time, we owe her so much. All BUPA's threats and bullying could not stop Private Eye printing our story for the first time. You can not sue for libel if the story is true. Thank God for private Eye they were brave enough to call BUPA's bluff. I started to realise that the truth could still prevail in spite of the law.

PRIVATE EYE. LESS THAN SUPER BUPA.

By Heather Mills.

While one of BUPA's directors, Des Kelly, has been advising Tony Blair on care of the elderly, a BUPA care home in Kent has been at the centre of grave allegations of abuse and neglect. Seven care workers who blew the whistle on a catalogue of cruelty, ill treatment, doping with sedatives and the withholding of drugs and treatment at the £322 a week Isard House in Bromley are due to be awarded compensation at an Employment Tribunal this week.

Except the seven-six women and one man-are boycotting the hearing and will refuse any payment from the U.Ks biggest private health insurer and care provider. The reason? The care workers say that though the Tribunal found in their favour, it so diluted or ignored serious allegations and evidence that neither they nor the vulnerable elderly they sought to protect-have received justice and they are challenging the tribunal's decision in court.

The care workers are outraged that BUPA continued to employ the women at the centre of the abuse against the subsequent advice of Social Services inspectors, at one stage trying to conceal the fact from them that she was working at a different vulnerable old peoples home. BUPA also promoted another who is to face further allegations from the daughter of a resident who has recently been removed from the home.

What concerned the Whistle-blowers most was while the Tribunal found it credible incontinent residents might not be changed quickly it did not find it credible they would be neglected to the extent they became filthy and sore, yet the whistle-blowers have the care plan of one resident showing that she had a sore that went to the bone. In another instance the Tribunal accepted the drugs sheet revealed the medication may not have been properly administered and or the recording was deficient, it ignored evidence suggesting records may have been falsified (The eye have examined several examples of the drug sheets, indicating they have been fabricated)

The seven whistle-blowers have asked The Lord Chancellors department to investigate their claims that dozens of pieces of evidence presented to the tribunal-in particular the evidence of independent witness's have been over looked.
They have also filed for Judicial review alleging

bias and misconduct on the part of the Tribunal saying they did not get a fair hearing. It could be argued that it is not the role of an Employment Tribunal to uncover levels of abuse, however as BUPA decided to brand the whistle-blowers as liars, they maintain the Tribunal should have evaluated all the evidence, hence their decision not to attend and try and block the compensation hearing.

Eileen Chubb told the eye "We can not fathom why BUPA would want to continue employing abusers, we went to court firstly for a declaration of the truth of what was going on in that home, and secondly for compensation, we will not accept any compensation, if the price to be paid is the truth."

Steve and I then had to assemble yet another set of the bundles for the high court, I filled in an application for judicial review and typed out a thirty page legal argument which referred to each piece of the evidence I relied on and stated the bundle, page and paragraph where it could be found.
I began to wonder what the lounge carpet looked like as I could not remember now it was always covered in bundles, witness statements and medical records.

Finally after ten days of hard slog, Steve and I went to London to deliver the bundles and lodge the case in the high court, we both nearly cried when the clerk told us we had to have two sets of everything, so we had no choice but to take all the bundles home again, photo copy everything and make yet another set of bundles.

Finally after another week of sorting hundreds of pages into order, hole punching and assembling a whole set of evidence bundles, we finished the extra set and went back to the high court weighed down with bundles and exhausted from the task of assembling them.

The clerk went through everything carefully as he knew we were not solicitors and I think he expected mistakes, we stood and watched him with baited breath for what felt like hours, I prayed they were right as I was so sick of assembling evidence bundles I thought I would scream if he said there was anything wrong with them. Finally the clerk said everything was in order and down came the official stamp of the court. When we got out side I stared at the official court forms for a moment and we both looked in awe at the words, The Royal Courts of Justice. "I hope it's true "I said "You hope what's true?" he asked and I said "That there really is justice in there like it says" We walked back to the train station our arms aching from the weight of the bundles we had delivered, but really amazed that we had done it and got this far with a £3.99 law book. I really needed to believe that someone would just look at the evidence if they did then they could not fail to see what had happened.

When I look back at those first court submissions I think they were not so bad. I laid it all out line by line as if I was trying to get an idiot to look at the blatantly obvious, no one could possibly have put it more clearly. I even cited precedents on the fear of the threat, which makes me smile because it came from Handsard and I thought then that Handsard was some bloke who had got the sack from his job, still the principle I was arguing was right and considering I had no idea what I was doing legally, I had something much more important then legal expertise. I had the absolute knowledge that I could prove what I was saying and could show any judge willing to look exactly where that proof was, I knew those bundles back to front. I no longer had a living room, a desk and fax machine were donated by well wishers. God, I thought that fax machine was the best thing since sliced bread. The post brought dozens of letters each day, box files and evidence bundles took up every spare inch of my once orderly house. The place looked like the campaign head quarters it had become. The phone never stopped ringing and I found people in the kitchen and had no idea when or how they had got there, it was like Piccadilly circus and the only reminders of the normal home life we used to have, were the television in one corner that we no longer had time to watch, and the book shelves in the other corner filled with the books we once had the time to read. The only thing I got to read anymore, were E.U Directives on Employment law, or the jurisdiction lists of Employment Tribunals.

A transformation was also taking place within me,

a transformation that would erase for ever the shy, easy going care assistant, I was no longer in awe of any one. It no longer occurred to me that I could not argue legal points with someone, just because they happened to be a judge or lawyer. I knew that what I was arguing for was right and if the law could not side with right, then it was no law at all.

Those around me saw the change long before I did, my dad once asked me where his daughter had gone, another old friend said "If there was a war I sure as hell would want to be on the same side as you" Which made me laugh but I was just too busy to stop and think about it. I think the first time it hit, just how much I had changed was after I came back from the high court, I suddenly thought "Where the hell did I go?"

Our first application to the high court was denied without a hearing on the grounds The Employment Appeal Tribunal, or E.A.T as they are referred to, were the remedy in our case. I made a renewal claim addressing these points and we were granted a hearing on June 20th 2002.
Steve and I had already done all the work that would normally be done by a solicitor, assembling the bundles, the court paperwork and submissions, serving the other parties and so on. But now we needed a barrister to speak for us in the high court just as we did at the Tribunal. A friend of a press contact asked a barrister they knew to telephone me and when he did call me he said," I know this is hard to believe but when it

comes to hearings for permission for judicial review, you actually stand a better chance if you speak yourself" he went on to say my submissions showed I knew the evidence better then anyone else could possibly learn it in time for the hearing. I was a bit panicked by this and asked him what I should say, he said that my submissions covered that already and that I should just summarise.

The day of the hearing came and Karen came with me to The Royal Courts of Justice, I had a case on wheels which I had packed with a spare set of the evidence bundles and the summery I was going to read out, we got to London very early to avoid any rushing and we had a coffee while we waited for the courts to open.

We were the first to arrive in the waiting area outside the courtroom, I thought it was the most impressive waiting room that I had ever seen with its stone floors and huge marble columns, even the heavy dark wood tables and chairs would not have looked out of place on the Antiques Road show. The whole building and everything in it felt very grand, very big so big that it made you feel very small and powerless in the might of all that legal history, overwhelmed by the grandeur of it all.

We sat down to wait, a large crowd arrived next, they were obviously all together and stood in a huddle talking in excited whispers, I recognised one of the women from the Ashford Tribunal, she was a solicitor from BUPA's in-house legal department.

There were several barristers in black robes and wigs, the only one of these I knew was Paul Epstein who I had thought at the time looked too experienced to be Laura Cox's junior. I had been right and had subsequently learnt he was a "Starvation Tactic" expert.

"Look" I said to Karen, "It's that Paul Epstein, do you think he would buy us a sandwich if I told him we were starving?" Other people started to slowly arrive in small groups of two or three, the other cases listed to be heard with ours I presumed. The court clerk came out and announced that everyone could go in to the court, and then he called out my name, "You are representing yourself?" I told him I was and he asked if I had ever been in a court before, I said only an Employment Tribunal. He said he would show me where to sit and explain the rules. Which he did as I followed him, he said there was ten cases in all and ours was listed last, "When each case is called the barrister will stand, when yours is called just put up your hand." I nodded I understood and looked around the huge dark wooden court room we had entered.

The clerk led me down some steep stairs and continued with his instructions. "You must address the judge as my lord and bow if he speaks to you and do not speak unless he gives you permission. Do not stand if you wish to speak hold up your hand, when he says you may speak only then may you do so but not before and do not forget to say, my lord and bow before you do. Have you got all that?" I said I understood him. He was a very nice man the clerk, he had a kind face and I think he was trying to help me as best he could. He left me sitting in what looked like a pit. I looked behind me and saw seats way up above me. Where all the barristers were now sitting, in front of me towering up above all else was a huge wooden wall, which was only broken by a bench half way up, where the kind faced clerk now sat, up above that the judges padded chair, empty as yet. There were only two other people in the pit with me, two middle aged men who I glanced at quickly. I thought they looked like they were waiting for sentence to be passed on them and I suddenly wondered if I was in the right place. This could be a dock I thought and I might get carted off to prison by mistake. The man closest to me must have noticed my worried look because he leaned forward, "First time?" he asked and when I nodded yes, he gave me what could only be described as a look of sincere condolence. Then the clerk got up and went up some steps at the side and disappeared for a moment, then returned and announced "All Rise" and in came the judge, who was tall, thin and looked a right misery. Mr Justice Lightman sat down and it did not take me long to conclude that justice was not his Christian name.

The name of the first case was called and I was thinking, it's going to be hours before they get to us. I looked around interested to see what the barrister was going to say, he bowed to the judge and had not even straightened up. When the judge barked "Permission denied" and the barrister had to bow himself backwards out of the room, "Blimey" I thought, "He must have had a bad case. "Then the next case was called and I looked around to see what was going to be said when "Permission denied" barked the judge and out bowed the barrister, I thought if this keeps up I may as well put my coat on. Two minutes later and six cases had been heard in the same way, God I thought you got the sentence after the hearing. It's the other way round here, the sentence being two words "Permission denied." Then the eighth case was called and yet another "permission denied" barked out. I held my breath when this young female barrister actually dared to speak "But my Lord the evidence", she actually managed to utter before the judge bellowed louder then ever through clenched teeth "I said permission is denied" and that was the end of that. One more bark of "permission denied" and our case was called and I thought he's not getting rid of me that easily I don't have to play by your rules and I forgot about being nervous and I no longer felt overwhelmed by the building. I just thought if that is justice than I will pay it the respect it's due. I stood up and politely but firmly launched into putting our case as quickly as I could.

"The E.A.T is the remedy for that" barked the judge, I calmly pointed out that the E.A.T had illegally denied our right to appeal. The judge looked like he did not believe me at all and barked at Paul Epstein. "Is what she saying right, I am not familiar with Employment Tribunal practice?" Then Paul Epstein who was supposed to be representing BUPA at their great expense got to speak for the first time and had to say "It would appear she is correct my Lord" the judge looked down at me and bellowed, "I have no copy of this ruling" and started banging the evidence bundles on his table while giving me looks that showed he thought it a dammed impertinence being made to look through evidence. I stayed calm and politely directed him to the relevant submissions listing the bundle and page number of the document in question. It was not long before he started banging the bundles on the bench again and shouted "I have no bundle three here." I still stayed calm and said I could oblige with a copy as I had brought a spare set of all the bundles submitted to the court in duplicate. I passed the bundle to the clerk who took it open mouthed and passed it up to the judge who banged it down on the table before looking at the document he wanted. I sat and waited while he read it and noticed he was madder then ever and his left eye had began to twitch as he bellowed, "Your bundles are too big anyway, they should only be that big", he held out his thumb and index finger and thrust them at me to emphasise his preferred size of bundle, being about an inch and a half. I wanted to tell him that I had only included the evidence Ashford had suppressed so it was their fault there was so much, but I kept calm and said "I see." I thought he looked like he was going to pop with the blood that seemed to be swelling his face so thought I had better go for it while I had a chance and launched into reading my summery as quickly as I could.

"The Ashford tribunal has shown clear prejudice in favour of the defendants, BUPA, not only in their findings of fact but in allowing the defendants BUPA change their witness statements after have sight of the applicant statements, and the statements of independent witness's, withholding evidence, allowing the applicants to be accused of criminal fraud in open court with no evidence to support this to boot, deferring the hearing when the defendants BUPA appealed, but refusing to defer the hearing when the applicants appealed. The applicants submit that the Public Interest Disclosure Act failed to protect them because the act is flawed, when the reasonable belief in disclosures is contested then those disclosures have to be judged. I submit that an Employment Tribunal is not qualified to judge criminal evidence, it therefore exceeded its jurisdiction and the applicant's right to a suitable qualified judge have been breeched and any remedy that does not comply with the natural laws of justice is no remedy at all.
I submit that the E.A.T is also firstly not qualified to judge criminal acts and secondly has shown clear prejudice in favour of the defendants BUPA, and the evidence upholds this. If the evidence for a time extension has been accepted by this court

then it is reasonable to expect it to be accepted by a lesser court. If the applicants case is denied on the grounds of being out of time then it is reasonable to expect that the defendants BUPA's objections also be denied if out of time.

The merit's of this case rests with the available evidence, which has been submitted in support of this case, we contest in full the findings of fact of the Ashford Tribunal and if the law is saying findings of fact can not be re judged then the law is saying that evidence can be suppressed and there is no remedy, the French declaration of the rights of man 1793 states "that any institution which does not suppose the people good and the magistrate corruptible is evil" We only ask that the law allows for such a possibility and provides a remedy.

The applicants claim the protection of the Human Rights Act and all articles and protocols therein (I had not read act yet, so was covering all angles) Furthermore the applicants claim the protection of all such rights and protocols in relation to those they sought to protect and we submit that we suffered a detriment as a direct result of seeing no reasonable steps being taken by the defendants BUPA, to protect the right to life and the right not to be tortured to those whom BUPA owed a duty of care.

What should not be forgotten is what lies at the heart of this case, the applicants were denied fair and just working conditions because they made disclosures relating to the inhuman treatment of defenceless elderly people, if the verdict of the

Beyond The Facade

Ashford Tribunal stands then so does the message it sends, The law will not protect you if you speak out against wrong in this country it's safer to look the other way, the evidence supports what has driven the applicants this far, what is right and true and the law that fails to uphold that fails to be a just law"

"HAVE YOU QUITE FINISHED NOW? Bellowed the judge, I had read the whole thing without drawing breath and was just about to say yes when up pipes Paul Epstein with "I really must object to the use of the word BUPA My..." "WHAT" bellows the judge who by this time was the colour of a blueberry and foaming at the mouth, I looked at the kind clerk who had a very expressive face and looked at me in exactly the same way he would have looked at someone, had they just run stark naked through the court and then he gave me a pitying smile, but it was I who felt sorry for him in truth as most of the judges saliva was landing on his head.

So the judge proceeds to spit out a ten minute judgement which included the fact that the EAT had denied us an appeal we had the right to, and that we could reapply on that point alone and have another hearing with Mr Lightman, the judge paused to glare down at me and he may as well have added, "if you have a death wish" for the look he gave me said it clearly, and then it was over, in all nearly an hour which was a dam sight more then the other poor sods got.

We walked out and heard BUPA whispering in a huddle, "They got what they came for", which was true in a way as I had to exhaust the legal remedy's here before we could take our case to Strasburg and Mr Justice Lightman was certainly exhausted.

We walked outside into the light and I took a deep breath, then I saw a man with a trolley piled high with thick bundles going into a side door, "Your going to bleeding cop it when they measure that lot" I said to him, he smiled at me in spite of looking puzzled and carried on by.

As we walked down the strand I turned to Karen and said "Contempt of court, I always wondered what that meant, how could you spend two minutes in that court, and fail to feel anything but contempt for it." It made me realise that it was bad enough fighting for this, but imagine having to depend on that legal system for your very liberty, I do not know what I expected in the High court, not much at all really after what the Tribunal had done to us, but I really wanted to believe there was such a thing as justice, I needed to believe that if justice existed then it would be found in that building. As we walked back to the train station I thought over everything that had happened and found myself wondering about something I had heard or read somewhere, the laws an ass or is it the laws an arse, I cant remember, I decided it must be an arse as it made more sense.

Beyond The Facade

I thought it could have been worse at least it only cost us a few pounds for a train ticket and I wondered how much those barristers had cost the poor sods who got only "Permission Denied" barked at them, at least I had got some time and I had gotten to speak. When I got home I told Steve what had happened and I did feel pleased that I had done my best, But I also felt sad, a kind of mourning I suppose for the country I thought I lived in, "Lets emigrate when this is all over, to some where more civilised like a banana republic" I said. We had already decided to go to Strasburg and the European Court of Human Rights should the high court refuse a hearing, not that we had any trust or expectation of justice in the legal system full stop, but because we felt we had to go on, there was no other way to bring BUPA to account so the abuse would stop. I think we all wanted someone to read the evidence and then we knew they would agree that the Ashford Tribunal had reached conclusions that were impossible to arrive at given the available evidence. I realised sometime later that we were fighting the legal system because it was part of the abuse. The Tribunal and the law were responsible for all the abuse that followed, because that is what protected the abusers. The Health Department were already sick of me and no minister would meet with me, they said they were too busy. In the end a senior civil servant agreed to meet with me, I arrived at The Health Department and the civil servant came down to meet me at the front desk and than took me up to his office. When I walked through the door I saw a large table spread with food and I felt a bit annoyed that he was obviously expecting someone for lunch and I would not be given much time, but he explained that the food was for me and I had plenty of time to tell him everything. He was a very nice man and was genuinely shocked, he assured me he would pass the information to a minister and than he said something I will never forget, "If this was America you would have been found floating down the river by now" and it was only later that I gave it any thought. Just before I left I asked for some of the leftover food to take home, after all it was a shame to waste it and I was pretty much shameless these days anyway. When I got home Steve asked me what I had got from them and I opened my bag and said "An apple two oranges and some breadsticks and a promise that a minister would be told about the case."

The best care company in the world could inadvertently employ abusers, the fact that abuse has taken place is not the test of a good company. The real test is what they do about it once they are informed of the abuse. If the stance of denial and cover-up is taken then that is what renders a care company unfit.

BUPA's denial and cover-up culture is so ingrained it goes to the very top. We were all told we could sue BUPA for slander for repeatedly calling us liars in the press, but that would have meant putting our trust in the law and it was the law that allowed BUPA to call us liars in the first place. So we fought on because we had no choice, if we gave up it was like saying the abuse was alright and we could not do that. A few days before we pleaded for the laws protection in the high court, Val Gooding C.B.E had gone on national television and called us liars yet again, she said that nothing of concern was ever found wrong at Isard House and that the Social Services inquiry report found no abuse, if the producer of the programme had not telephoned me prior to the interview they would never have seen a copy of this report, fortunately I was able to fax them a copy in time so Val Gooding could at least be challenged on this.

BBC HARDTALK 14th Of June 2002.

Transcripts of interview with Val Gooding.

Q. What about care for the elderly, why is it that the elderly are often abused in health care homes?

Val Gooding. "I don't know where you get that impression, that they are often abused, I think the standards in this country are very high on the whole. There are issues in care for the elderly, mainly in the area of funding, there is inadequate funding for care of the elderly and there has been numerous attempts to try and right this situation, but never the less care homes are still closing"

Q. Seven hundred and fifty homes closed last year, it's a major issue for the public, is it not, care of the elderly?

Val Gooding. "Yes it is a major issue and I think it's a major issue for all of us, we have parents who are elderly and eventually we will be elderly ourselves, who is going to look after us and how is it going to be paid for and I think this is a very big question for the country as a whole"

Q. is it a bad sign if seven hundred and fifty homes closed last year?

Val Gooding. "Indeed and the only reason really that they closed is the economics are not good, it is very hard for single operators to make a return, many operators have sold their homes because they can make more money out of them as property, by converting them back to property"

Q. BUPA is not immune itself from allegations that people have suffered abuse in your homes, there was one in West Riding, a nursing home, nurses ignored a pensioners screams of pain after she fell and broke her leg, a patient left for five hours, how do you feel about that?

Beyond The Facade

Val Gooding "Occasionally things can go wrong but we have extremely high standards of supervision, of training and of inducting our employees into our care home environment, we have very high quality control standards, if something does go wrong and things will go wrong occasionally, we always investigate them thoroughly, if necessary we will retrain the person concerned, on the whole incidents are very rare"

Q. Did the Isard house in Bromley, which is another home run by you, allegations were made in 1999, did that live up to your high standards?

Val Gooding "Indeed, absolutely"

Q. The care lived up to your high standards?

Val Gooding "Absolutely, we never found anything remiss about that home"

Q. The Bromley team did though? They upheld a complaint made by the Whistle-blowers, who brought the case to the Authorities attention?

Val Gooding "That is not correct, Bromley Social Services on whose behalf we run that home are still entirely satisfied in the way that home is run, there are no issues outstanding at all"

Q. Even though the inspection team said that the team leader was primarily responsible for allowing the climate of abusive and neglectful behaviour to exist unchecked?

Val Gooding "There is no substantiation to that claim what so ever, nothing"

Q. Your own Clair Cater who said last year, she admitted there were issues which were wrong in one unit, she said steps were being taken to correct them?

Val Gooding "There was one issue, which was about the recording of medication, nothing to do with abuse what so ever"

Q. The other allegations of abuse, repeated physical abuse, drugs deliberately withheld and other drugs given without prescription?

Val Gooding "All of these have been thoroughly investigated by, the police, the industrial Tribunal, by Social Services and not least by ourselves, because we were determined to get to the bottom of these issues, nothing substantive was found at all. Bromley Social Services still give us their business, they are entirely satisfied with the way that home is run"

Q. Clair Cater said last year on behalf of your company, she found some exaggeration in a few of the allegations but she accepted they had been made in good faith, she also admitted one member of staff had panicked and tried to hide the fact that the team leader was re-deployed else where?

Val Gooding "It's always very difficult is it not, in these situations to know which member of staff is giving an accurate version of events and there was some of these issues surrounding this particular incident, what I have to do is, I have to be confident that we are looking after vulnerable people well and we are and I am confident about that"

Q. But we can not have allegations like this being made and being left for a long time before action is taken?

Val Gooding "No not at all, never, and I do sometimes think we make mistakes in not following up something quickly enough or what ever but that is not the culture of our company, the culture of our company is to investigate any allegations immediately and act on it, if we have any cause for concern, in this case we have none"

I rang the local papers and they covered the story about the Val Gooding interview so it was at least a small consolation as we could defend ourselves and respond to her calling us liars. I did feel angry with those in Bromley Council who had renewed BUPA's contract as it allowed BUPA to say the Council were happy with the way they were running the homes. I started writing letters to all of Bromley's Councillors and the Director of Social

Services, and asked them if they were willing to take responsibility for any more abuse happening. At first they replied with assurances that no more abuse would occur as BUPA were complying with all the recommendations in the inquiry report. The very report that BUPA disputed in the Tribunal and that Val Gooding dismissed so casually.

THE KENTISH TIMES. 21/6/02

BUPA CHIEFS RUBBISH ABUSE ALLEGATIONS.

In April Bromley Council extended BUPA's contract to run six homes in the borough for two years on the recommendation of DAVID ROBERTS, Bromley's Assistant Director for older people, he said "If BUPA had not been up to the job it would have been dealt with eighteen months ago in the investigation, we have tightened up the monitoring at Isard House and it appears to be working"

I bombarded Bromley's Director of Social Services, Jeremy Ambache, with letters of concern and I sent copies of each one of these letters and the replies I received to every member of the Social Services committee. If I was not typing letters then I was addressing envelopes, reading inspection reports or sat in council meetings taking notes. The Director of Social

Services, Jeremy Ambache went sick and the local paper covered his retirement.

THE BROMLEY EXPRESS 15/5/02

By R.T Quayle.

The resignation of Bromley's Social Services Director has not come as a surprise to all in the beleaguered department. Jeremy Ambache quit after just two years in the post, Bromley council accepted with immediate effect his application for early retirement. Malcolm Hyland, retiring chairman of Bromley's Social Services Committee, said" The work needed to remedy large scale problems within the service could have persuaded Mr Ambache to bow out."
His resignation is the latest in a series of big name departures from Social Services.
Social Services has been long dogged by high profile inquiries into allegations of abuse at Betts way in Penge and Isard House in Bromley.

Less than twelve weeks after I was assured by Bromley Council that there would be no more abuse, another story was covered by the local paper, Audrey Ford had died and a coroners inquest was held to examine the circumstances of her death, after this evidence was considered the Coroner recorded an open verdict on the grounds that the Anti-psychotic drugs administered in Isard

House could not be discounted as causing death. Bromley Council refused to comment when I asked them if they were still confident in BUPA's fitness to manage their care homes.

THE NEWSHOPPER. 16/10/2002

DID SHE DIE NEEDLESSLY?

By Richard Simcox.

Last week a Coroner was unable to say whether 83 year old Audrey Fords death was caused by her illness or by the Anti Psychotics drugs she had been prescribed, the open verdict effectively bolsters seven BUPA whistle-blowers taking their case to Europe.

So once more Steve and I assembled yet another set of bundles, the court paperwork was filled out and submissions cross referencing the evidence typed out, the more courts we went through the more paperwork accumulated and we had a bundle on just the legal remedies we had tried alone. Finally it was ready and packed into a large box and it all went of to Strasburg and we waited and hoped yet again. But by now I knew it would take a miracle for a judge to actually read the evidence and the evidence was everything. We had not built our case on legal argument that twisted the law to suit our needs, our case rested on the evidence which proved beyond any doubt that the Ashford's Tribunals suppression of this evidence was not lawful, the submissions I wrote explained and guided any one willing to turn the pages, it was just a matter of finding some one who was willing to do that.

I met a barrister through another persons case and I explained where we were with our case, "The trouble is" he said "No subsequent court will ever examine the evidence to the degree of the court who first heard it."
I knew that in my heart but it seemed so wrong that a judge could make things up or suppress vital evidence and not be answerable to anyone, I suppose that's why they feel they can get away with doing such things in the first place. I remembered people being really shocked by the verdict in the Hutton Inquiry, I was not shocked at all, I had sat in far too many courts, and by that time had seen far too much injustice to be shocked that a judge could do what Lord Hutton did, just because a judge said it, you can not presume it to be true. I remembered what the man in the Health Department had said to me about been found floating down the river and wondered if woods were not the preferred sites for whistle-blowers to be found in this country. It's my experience that you are more likely to find people of a higher moral code in Wormwood Scrubs than sitting in judgement in Courts and Tribunals. It took nearly a year before we got a letter from

Eileen Chubb

Strasburg saying a judge would look at our case the following Thursday afternoon. It would have taken at least a week to actually read the evidence, so when we received a single sentence letter stating we had not pursued our remedies here, it was to us just one more slap in the face from the law that had betrayed us from the outset, Linda Clark said when I told her the news from Strasburg, "Wouldn't it have been really something if we had got justice in spite of law." I thought that pretty much summed up the law really.

It's small wonder to me that the Human Rights Act, is now held in such contempt, when you consider how it has been twisted by lawyers to suit the needs of the few, whilst those in need of its protection the most, the vulnerable victims abused in care, have no rights, not even the right to life itself.

I do not know what it's like at Guantamino Bay, perhaps the prisoners have burnt and bruised bodies like those I saw in Isard House. Perhaps they too are subjected to constant physical and physiological torture, like that I witnessed in Isard House and if that is so than it shames us all. But what shames us even more is that Guantamino Bay makes the news and human rights lawyers are willing to represent those held there, and while we hold up our hands in horror at Guantamino Bay. In the care home down the road elderly people are subjected to the most horrific suffering, torture and stripped of all human rights and for the crime of being old, and when against all the odds this abuse is brought out into the open. The law in this civilised country of ours looks the other way.

Edna and those like her are invisible, their suffering is called anything other then abuse and torture so that it can be made acceptable, well shame on the Government, The law, and BUPA for they are all worse by far then the Maria Keenahan's of this world. Those elderly people at the mercy of what we ironically call a "care system", fought to make this country what it is. I for one will not stand by and see them stripped of all rights, I have seen the face of suffering and heard it's cries, when I was in Isard house I wanted to run round shouting "Sanctuary" I still do.

KENT ON SUNDAY 5/9/04

By Jamie McGinnes.

Shadow Home Secretary David Davis has backed a call from a group of former caseworkers to bring in better safeguards for Whistle-blowers.
Mr Davis encouragement came as the BUPA seven hit back at their former employers dismissal of their claims of patient mistreatment. In an earlier article in the Kent on Sunday BUPA said "It encouraged Whistle-blowers to come forward" but Mrs Chubb said "She would feel safer informing on the Mafia" and she refuted BUPA's assertion that none of the concerns raised in 1999 were ever substantiated, she showed the Kent on

Eileen Chubb

Sunday a copy of a report by Bromley Social Services which upheld allegations about patient care at Isard House. But peter Ludford, Director of BUPA Care homes this week dismissed the findings of the report claiming that any failings identified were only "Minor."

Every time BUPA issued a press statement the denial got worse, I thought I was beyond being shocked by what they said, but I remember when the reporter rang me and said they are calling the findings "Minor" I was shocked, it's such a small insignificant word to justify so much suffering, I told the reporter it was hardly surprising that abuse was still happening when you considered what BUPA thought to be minor.

PRIVATE EYE, 3/8/04.

By Heather Mills.

BUPA finally seems to be getting to grips with the serious problems relating to the care of old people that have dogged Isard House care home in Bromley for the last five years. Since the eye last appeared more staff at the home have been sacked or suspended amid allegations of mistreatment and neglect, following the arrival of a hit squad from BUPA, investigations are continuing and more disciplinary action is expected. One sacked care worker is understood to have been one of those whom BUPA relied on five years ago to defend itself against claims from seven whistle-blowers of serious abuse and neglect in the home, which caters for up to 66 old people with high levels of dependency, it was alleged residents had been left in their own mess, were handled roughly and inappropriately drugged.

More recently reports from the new Commission for Social Care Inspection, have failed to spot the issues currently at the centre of allegations at the home, but the commission has found that the home has consistently failed to reach even the minimum standards in care needs and training. It also expressed concern about the high numbers of falls and accidents requiring hospital treatment. Yesterday BUPA declined to give any details of the latest allegations, but said it was continuing to investigate "Concerns raised by staff." To date five disciplinary hearings are due to take place, one staff member has been dismissed and one has been given a written warning. Eileen Chubb one of the original whistle-blowers said "The trouble is that by denying and fighting our claims five years ago, BUPA sent the wrong message to the core of the staff at the home and because of that, nothing has changed." She may be right, advertisements have already appeared in the local paper for an unspecified number of staff, phoning up to enquire about a job as a senior care worker, an eye reporter was offered an immediate interview, she was not asked about any previous experience, qualifications, or if she had a criminal record, all mentioned as areas of concern in the last inspection report.

The law would not help us so that only left the political process and Lord Falconer can confirm I took that to the limits. I wrote hundreds of letters to Government Departments and they tied themselves in knots trying to fob me off onto any other Department but theirs.

Lord Falconer said the D.T.I were responsible for the Public Interest Disclosure Act.
So I asked the D.T.I who was responsible for judging criminal disclosures,
The D.T.I said the proscribed regulator was responsible.
I asked the D.T.I who was the prescribed regulator under the law, for abuse in care homes,
The D.T.I said Social services inspection,
I asked the D.T.I why the Tribunal had ignored the regulator and judged the criminal disclosures
The D.T.I said ask Lord Falconers Department.
So I asked Lord Falconer who responded with "No comment"
So I asked Lord Falconer if our case could not be heard in, An Employment Tribunal, the E.A.T or the High Court, then which court could hear it.
Lord Falconer was unable to say, and that was a summery of an average week of correspondence.
The campaign continued and was well covered by the press.

Beyond The Facade

THE NEWSHOPPER 23/7/04

by Richard Simcox.

*M.P calls for an inquiry over the BUPA Seven
Case.*

*Ministers are being pressed to hold a full public
inquiry into the case of seven former caseworkers
fighting to protect Whistle-blowers. Orpington M.P
John Horam called on colleagues to urge the
Government to investigate the case of the, "BUPA
Seven" members claim they were forced to leave
their jobs after alleging abuse at a BUPA run
home five years ago. "Workers not speaking out is
a major contributory factor in elder abuse in care
homes" a petition presented to the House of
Commons by Mr Horam last Thursday says.
The campaigners want the Department for
Constitutional Affairs to review the 1998, Public
Interest Disclosure Act, but the Newshoppers
inquiries to the D.C.A were directed to the Health
Department who said "It was too early to say
whether a public inquiry would be held", but that
the petition would be, "Looked Into."
Director of BUPA care services, Peter Ludford,
said "The concerns raised by the former
caseworkers have been exhaustively investigated
by the Police, CPS and heard at an Employment
Tribunal, none found sufficient evidence to support
claims of ill treatment of residents, BUPA have
robust whistle-blowing policies in place."*

I wrote to Lord Falconer and reminded him that to date, he held the Public Interest Disclosure to be the responsibility of the D.T.I, the D.T.I said it's Lord Falconers responsibility and when a News reporter asks he is sent to the Health Department. It's no surprise this legislation is such a shambles when no one even knows whose responsible for it. On the end of every news article the usual denial from BUPA and I felt angry every time BUPA said the police had investigated and found nothing wrong, I knew that could not have happened but I could not prove it.

THE NEWSHOPPER. 1/11/04.

By Richard Simcox.

Campaigners battling the British legal system donned wigs and gowns to take their fight to Westminster, dressed as law lords Eileen Chubb and Karen Hook met Orpington M.P John Horam at the House of Commons. Joined by fellow, BUPA Seven members and supporters, they handed over letters addressed to all MPs and Peers calling for the law protecting so called Whistle-blowers to be tightened.
What started out as an Employment Tribunal in 1999 has escalated into a full scale assault on the Government.
Joyce earl secretary of the Bromley branch of the, British Pensioners Trade Union said," What

saddens us is knowing there are so many careworkers turning a blind eye to such injustices shown towards people who have few ways of defending themselves." Mr Horam said, "The principles they are trying to get established are important, they have had a raw deal that is why we need a proper law". BUPA said they "Considered the matter closed."

We prepared to go to meet John Horam and handover the letters for the MPs and peers, I had decided to use one of the recent letters I had written to Lord Falconer, as it was a good example of all the key points in our case. I thought I would never finish typing all the envelopes and we had a conveyor belt going when it came to folding the letters and sealing the envelopes, which we had to use a wet sponge to do before long, as licking the gummed edges was making us feel sick. Finally we packed over a thousand letters into two suitcases on wheels, we then photo copied over two thousand information leaflets and forms for the public to send to their MPs.

There was only a few days left before we went to London and I thought we may as well make the most of the opportunity and dress up. I thought Judges summed up what we were fighting, so Karen made two judges gowns out of some curtains and we bought two wigs, which were so hot to wear that we nearly passed out.
I found I had a talent for slogans so I thought up

some and typed them out and had them enlarged and someone kindly lent us a laminator, Steve and I made placards, hole punched and threaded string through so they could be worn like a sandwich board, one on the front and another on the back, leaving the hands free, "In case we need to chain ourselves to any railings" I joked. But really it was because a lot of our supporters were elderly and I did not want them to have to carry heavy placards.

We had things like "Justice for the BUPA Seven" and "The Law takes the pea out of Whistle-blowers" and plenty of other slogans. I made up special placards for myself and Karen to wear over our judges robes, "The law says it's alright to kick a defenceless old women" and then we had a smaller sign lower down in a suitable place to emphasise the message which said, "The Law my arse."

The morning of the protest came and people started to arrive and the house was packed by the time Karen and I went into my bedroom to put on our judges outfits. Just before we left the house I caught a glimpse of myself in a mirror for the first time and it suddenly hit me that I was about to get on a train for London in the rush hour, looking like a cross between judge John Deed and Lily Savage, I knew right then why people climbed buildings dressed as batman, they were driven to it by a government who refused to listen. Well if this is what it takes then so be it, I thought and we set off for the train station stopping the traffic all the way.

When we got on the train for London that day, I saw something that made up for all the unjust judges, indifferent politicians and corrupt care companies, as soon as the general public saw our placards we were overwhelmed by offers of support, the whole of the train carriage asked for information and forms for their MPs. I will always remember the young Australian lad that was sitting next to me, he said he was staying with friends so he had no M.P but his mates had and he asked if he could have some information, he started to read the leaflet and was half way down the page when he shouted loudly, "Strewth, God almighty is that true?" When I said it was the words of the court he said, "That's a bloody disgrace" and he asked for a pile of forms for everyone he worked with, out of all the people I met that day it's that young lad I remember most, it was not that he surprised me by saying, "Strewth", when I never thought Australians really said that, it was not because of the look of absolute horror on his face, I remembered him most because he was so willing to read the pages when no judge had been willing to do the same. By the time we reached Charring Cross we had handed out over a thousand letters and forms. I had looked up at one point, and saw queues stretching as far as I could see, people came down from all the other carriages. I felt the tears well up and lowered my eyes quickly and continued handing out the forms. I felt humbled by how much people cared and for the first time in a long time, I felt proud of the country I lived in. That same support continued all of that day, as we walked to Westminster people stopped and offered their support. The traffic was tooting us, it was the London cabbies who were the funniest, constantly we heard shouts of, "The bleeding laws a disgrace" "good for you" and "Them bleeding judges ought to be locked up if you ask me."

When we arrived outside the House of Commons a burley Policeman descended on us looking furious," You can not demonstrate here the house is sitting, who's in charge?" he demanded, everyone pointed at me whilst staring at the gun the Policeman held, "It's OK"I said "We are not demonstrating, we have an appointment with John Horam M.P and it's about this" and I handed him one of our leaflets and he went off for a couple of minutes, when he came back he did not look quite so stern, "Just stand there and behave and we will presume you always dress like that" he said and gave a quick smile before walking off. Just standing there was enough, with me and Karen as bookends, people formed orderly queues behind us to read our placards and then asked for leaflets. The Japanese tourists wanted to pay us to have a photograph taken with them, we declined the money but let them take pictures," We should have done this instead of them boot sales", said Linda.

Beyond The Facade

John Horam arrived, the press came and took photos and the nice Policeman called out to his colleagues" You can't see this for two minutes" as the photographs were taken just a little bit too close to the entrance. We handed over to Mr Horam the sacks of letters and he took them into the house, I had to go with him to the commons post room and have the sacks x-rayed by security and then we all went to a pub nearby for a cup of tea and when the pub landlord saw what Karen and I had on our backs and he told us to sit with our backs to the wall," Judges come in here you know" he said in an outraged tone.

NEWSHOPPER 11/03

By Richard Simcox.

A Barrister is backing calls for better protection for Whistle-blowers, Patrick Green who specialises in Employment law, says legislation has only been a "Good First Step" in a radio interview he said the Public Interest Disclosure Act does not go far enough in protecting those raising" Serious Issues" in the public interest. Mr Green was interviewed on BBC radio fours, You and yours programme along side Orpington M.P John Horam, who is calling for a public inquiry into the battle waged by seven former care workers to bolster the act. Last week Newshopper reported how Eileen Chubb and supporters delivered letters to all MPs and Peers asking for support.

I kept writing letters by the dozen and wrote to all the unions and the heads of professional bodies asking for their support, I was always amazed and heartened by how quickly that support was offered.

NEWSHOPPER 10/12/03.

By Richard Simcox.

High profile support is mounting for a campaign to tighten up the law protecting so called "Whistle-blowers."
Now former care workers who are lobbying the Lord Chancellor Lord Falconer, to strengthen the Public Interest Disclosure act have the support of senior doctors.
In a letter to campaigner Eileen Chubb, Hospital Consultants and Specialists Association Chief Executive, Stephen Campion writes, "I wish your campaign success in highlighting deficiencies in the system"

My workload was massive, every day the post brought dozens of letters and every evening that days work would be posted, I had a list of who needed phoning and a message book to record the constant incoming calls, the photo copier was going constantly, every night there was a huge pile of reading to be got through.

I remembered as a child seeing this man at the circus who had all these plates spinning on poles and he would run up and down trying to keep all the plates spinning and had just got to the end of the line when he would have to run back to the beginning and start all over again, I felt like just like that man only if I stopped it would be more than plates that got broken, so I kept going.

NEWSHOPPER.

By Richard Simcox.

Union members are calling for national support for a campaign to tighten up the law protecting Whistle-blowers. The Transport and General Workers Union branch representing pensioners is backing the BUPA Sevens battle with the law. National Union of Journalists General Secretary Jeremy Dear also "Fully endorses" the fight for reform of the law. BUPA Director Peter Ludford said "It is vital to recognise the importance of Whistle-blowing."

Lord Falconer had not been able to defend the laws treatment of our case, in fact he had tried every conceivable excuse to avoid addressing the questions our case raised, as often the way with politicians, he tried to change the subject, in the end he was reduced to saying no comment. So we organised a protest outside Lord Falconers Department For Constitutional Affairs.

Again we sat off for London dressed as Judges, we asked anyone who was able to support us to meet us at Charring Cross Train Station. We were again overwhelmed by support on the train and when we arrived at Charring Cross and stepped of the train I heard a lot of shouting from a large crowd somewhere nearby, I turned to the others and said, "Oh no there's a load of hooligans and we are dressed like this" and then I caught sight of who was making all the noise "Oh God their our hooligans" I said, people had come from all over to support us, from the Bromley pensioners union to The Lynde House relatives Association and my dear friend Gillian Ward had dressed as an undertaker and wore a large notice which said, The death of justice.

It was freezing cold that day and all these people stood with us all day outside Lord Falconers Department, we sang songs, handed out leaflets and talked to the public. I had written a special song about our case, the tune was taken from an old Music Hall song and I changed the words,

Beyond The Facade

The BUPA Seven Song.

For being honest we now are poor,
For speaking of their cruel fate
Because we tried to protect the elderly,
BUPA chucked us out the gate.

It's the law the whole world over
Aint it just a blooming shame
It's the innocent what is punished
Whilst the guilty gets no blame.

For those who blow the whistle
The law is doomed to fail,
But the truth cannot be hidden,
For our silence aint for sale.

It's the law the whole world over
Aint it just a blooming shame,
It's the innocent what is punished
Whilst the guilty gets no blame.

The world would be much better,
If injustice were a crime
But we'd have to build more prisons
For all them judges serving time.

It's the same the whole world over,
Aint it just a blooming shame
It's the innocent what is punished
Whilst the guilty gets no blame.

Lord Falconer he is mighty

But the mighty can fall as well
And if he thinks that we will falter
He aint got an hope in hell.

It's the same the whole world over,
Aint it just a blooming shame
It's the innocent what is punished
Whilst the guilty gets no blame.

Twas the case of the BUPA Seven
That proved the law is just a farce
And if that's what they call justice
They can poke it up their arse.

Repeat chorus.

It brought the house down as crowds gathered to
listen, cheering and applauding it brought more
people and they all asked for more information,
which this time we had enough supplies of to meet
the demand, we had gone with five thousand
information sheets and returned with not a single
one. We met loads of really lovely people that day
and everyone was really cheered by the response
we got from the public, it made us forget how cold
and dismal the weather was. We handed in a
letter to Lord Falconer and later received the
response "No comment."

Joyce Earl from the pensioners union suggested
that I write to Tony Benn, so I did and asked him
how I could get our case heard in Parliament, he

was very helpful and told me how to petition the Government through the House of Commons.

I wrote out the first of two petitions according to the rules and my M.P John Horam read it out in parliament on the 15th of July 2004 at 6.13pm.

Handsard.

"I wish to present a petition on behalf of Eileen Chubb of the BUPA Seven, the BUPA Seven is composed of former care workers who spoke out against elder abuse in a care home in Bromley, the petition states,
That silence is a major contributory factor in elder abuse in care homes and that unless Whistle-blowers are protected, the silence will continue, along with the suffering of those who are unable to speak out for themselves, the petitioners further declare that the case of the BUPA Seven, has raised real concerns that the Public Interest Disclosure Act is failing to protect those who speak out in the legitimate interest of others, amongst these failings is the fact that if the employer contests the disclosures then the Whistle-blower is left in a situation where the only court who can hear the evidence has no jurisdiction to hear criminal evidence. The petitioners further declare that the verdict in the case of the BUPA Seven will serve to encourage others not to report abuse and they note the conclusions of the Health Select Committee report

*on elder abuse that further measures to make staff
aware of their responsibility to report abuse and to
allow them to do this in a confidential manner are
needed.*

The Governments official response "No comment"

The Freedom of Information Act came into force
and the first thing I did was make a request to both
the Police and The C.P.S for all the case files on
the investigation they carried out, only when I
received these files did I have the proof that no
investigation had been carried out at all.
I had the records of every action the Police had
ever taken and those records showed that not only
was no witness ever interviewed but neither was
any suspect, from the time I arrived at the Police
station with the evidence bundles, to the time the
Police decided there was no prospect of a
prosecution was all of forty minutes. I took the
records to Heather Mills at Private Eye.
(Extract below, see index for full story)

Private Eye 4/3/05, BUPA DON'T CARE HOMES.

By Heather Mills.

*Former care staff who made serious allegations of
neglect, potentially fatal doping and mistreatment
of old people at Isard House, a BUPA run care
home near Bromley in Kent, have at last learned*

what action police took in response to a dossier of evidence they submitted three years ago, it was all but ignored.

No statement was taken from any witness, no member of staff from the home was interviewed and BUPA it's self was never even approached over the allegations. In fact police notes suggest that just a few hours after three bundles of documents, mainly complex medical records were submitted officers had already decided that "No crime had been confirmed."

This is alarming since on face value the medical sheets seemed to show that a number of elderly residents were given potentially fatal doses of powerful drugs. One resident E.P (Edna) had on four occasions been given a dose of tranquilliser that was Nine times the daily prescribed dose, 30mls and Six times higher then what is considered safe for an elderly person. Eye readers may also recall the case of Audrey Ford another Isard House resident who was taken to hospital suffering from the side-effects of a powerful Anti psychotic which should only have been given to those suffering severe mental illness, like Schizophrenia. She never recovered and the Coroner recorded an open verdict

The deluge by post of all MPs continued and than I found out what had been going on in Isard House and the other BUPA homes in Bromley since the time we were forced out of our jobs. Whilst we had waited for first the law and then the Government to act and despite all the huge efforts that were made, the abuse had continued.

THE NEWSHOPPER. 13/7/05

By Bede McGowan.

Whistle-blowers are calling for the resignation of a Social Services chief after a damming report was published into care standards at six BUPA homes, Shaw Healthcare took over the running of Bromley's care homes for the elderly in April 05, when the councils contract ran out. Since the transfer 280 staff have undertaken a training program on skills such as, the administration of medication, adult protection and whistle-blowing. Members of the BUPA Seven resigned as caseworkers from Isard house in 1999, alleging abuse as well as potentially fatal drugging of elderly people.
Spokesman Eileen Chubb said "The care failings listed in this report show elderly vulnerable people have suffered for six years and that suffering was totally avoidable, we now call for DAVID ROBERTS resignation." Mr Roberts declined to comment…BUPA have always said there was no evidence to support the BUPA Sevens allegations, a BUPA spokesman said "We strongly refute any suggestion that the new provider inherited poor quality care."

Beyond The Facade

Finally even Bromley Council reached its limit, enough people had been abused for them to take some action, and BUPAS contract was not renewed and only than did some of the suffering come to light. However David Roberts who had previously extended BUPAS contract refused to resign, again there is no accountability for abuse, it's only ever the victims who pay the price.

THE KENT ON SUNDAY. 17/7/05

WHISTLE-BLOWERS VINDICATED

By Jamie McGinnes.

Whistle-blowers say they have been vindicated by a damming report into care homes, a meeting of Bromley Social care Committee was told that standards have improved at six care homes since BUPA stopped managing them. Eileen Chubb told the Kent on Sunday, "This report now vindicates us, we will continue to fight for justice until those in positions of authority acknowledge we were always telling the truth and that the abuse was saw inflicted on defenceless elderly people was wrong, what saddens us the most is we ever had to fight for this in the first place"....
The report said, "Shaw healthcare have dealt robustly with incidents of poor quality care, additionally Shaw healthcare has tackled individual issues in conjunction with CSCI through

Eileen Chubb

its disciplinary procedures."
*Eileen Chubb said "how can a new provider inherit
care staff that requires disciplinary action? If Shaw
healthcare can see these problems within weeks
of taking over, surely BUPA must also have been
aware of them"*
BUPA Deny all the allegations.

PRIVATE EYE. 16/7/05.

By Heather Mills.

*Isard House, Bromley councils report on the
successful transfer of six of it's care homes from
BUPA to Shaw, makes very interesting reading,
the homes included Isard House where seven
Whistle-blowers lost their jobs after making
allegation of abuse, drugging and ill-treatment,
The report said one of the major areas of concern,
the large numbers of admissions to hospital of
elderly people through falls and ill-health had"
Significantly reduced." This is good news for the
residents as it was as long ago as 19999 that the
BUPA Whistle-blowers lost their jobs, ever since
they have had to fight tooth and nail to get the
council and BUPA to act on their claims, the
council put out the contract to tender last year,
BUPA however remains in denial, spokesman
Oliver Thomas said "We strongly refute any
suggestion that the new provider inherited poor
quality care, the regulators were always satisfied*

with the care we provided."

I continued to make use of The Freedom of Information Act and sent inquests left right and centre, one of the reports I unearthed was about how many people had falls and injuries. I had by now established a good routine that worked on three basis principles, firstly get the information, then assess that information and finally make sure the public know what it's in their interest to know, the press were brilliant in helping me achieve the latter.

KENT ON SUNDAY 1/5/05

By Jamie McGinnes.

A private healthcare firm has apologised over new figures appeared to show the number of falls at a care home it ran where higher then previously suggested. BUPA which ran the home until last month had maintained there were only 16 night time "Accidents", but a newly unearthed report shows there were 34 night time falls in that period alone. Eileen Chubb requested the figures from Bromley council under the new, Freedom of Information Act. Mrs Chubb said she was disturbed to read minutes of a meeting between BUPA and Bromley council, which detailed an incident where a frail old women at Isard house was found with a broken arm one morning in February 2004, in the minutes the manager of the home complained that staff had been found sleeping on duty. However this incident does not appear in the fall statistics for Jan to July 2004. Terry Rich director of Social Services said he did not want to comment on the falls figures saying that CSCI carry out regular inspections at Isard House.

I got used to being in the newspapers, there were stacks of press cuttings on the BUPA Seven case and I found it very easy to work with the media, I did loads of T.V and radio also but the one that I will always remember was the first T.V programme I ever did, it was Kilroy, I walked onto the set and saw my name on a seat right at the front, I had expected to be sitting far back in the audience and that was nerve racking enough but sitting there at the front I felt so exposed, not to mention my tatty shoes could be seen by all.

I reluctantly went and sat in the allotted place and almost immediately a man came over and said I would be wearing a microphone and asked me to thread the wire up through my top, he then clipped it on my collar and walked off with the rest of the lead. I felt like I had been strapped into the chair, which was just as well as when the music came on and this camera started to loom in on me, the only thing that stopped me bolting out of there was the thought I was plugged into some expensive sound equipment and if I ran it would blow up like the final scene in a James Bond Movie.

I felt blind panic and froze staring at the camera like a rabbit in a cars headlights. I do not know what exactly happened after that until this politician said something so stupid that I completely forgot where I was and I snapped out of my panic, I turned to him and put him straight about his ignorance. The politician looked like he wanted to kill me and after that I never shut up, when it was over they said it would be broadcast next day and I could not remember a word I had said by the time I got home.

By the next morning I was convinced that I had made a complete fool of myself on national television, I sat down to watch the programme holding a large cushion, ready to bury me head in shame. I could hardly believe it was me speaking, I did not even recognise my own voice at first, I heard the absolute determination that I had felt for so long come through, when the programme finished the phone started ringing "I bet they will never put another politician on the same show as you after that" my mum said.

The applicants press officer they jokingly called me. I felt like I had always worked with the media it came naturally, the media were our only chance of getting the truth out. I did so much T.V and radio it became routine, you could just about fit a camera and sound crew and all their equipment into our tiny flat, but we packed them in. I remember once recording a BBC File on Four programmes, the producer was doing a sound check in the living room and our dog who was a puppy took a dislike to the microphone and kept trying to kill it, so Steve had to stand in the hall with the dog on a lead and wait with the shows presenter.

Steve told me afterwards he needed the loo and had to ask the presenter to hold the dog for a minute, "You cant even go to the toilet in this house without the BBC knowing about it "he said, I laughed as it pretty much summed up the mad house we now lived in.

My biggest achievement in press coverage happened one evening, we were being filmed for a BBC Documentary called, Britain's Secret Shame, whilst we were listening to a radio broadcast that I recorded the week before and the local papers sent photographers to take pictures of us being filmed as we listened to our case on the radio, it was absolute chaos and no one noticed the dog eating all the sandwiches in the background.

I was filmed empting dustbins at my cleaning job, walking in the park, posting letters, making tea, and once I was filmed doing a reconstruction of the day I went to the Civic Centre to report the abuse, Dickon the BBC cameraman was very particular and I had to walk into the Civic Centre over a dozen times before he was happy with the footage, after I had walked in the first couple of times, the receptionists noticed and started to watch each time I came through the doors and turned and walked out again, they could not see the cameraman and must have thought I was some kind of lunatic with a fetish for automatic doors, going by the looks they gave me.

When we came out of the high court in the summer of 2002, we did not know that the abuse that was continuing at Isard house would eventually be made public, but we knew that the abuse continued, how could it not when BUPA encouraged it to thrive in a climate of secrecy and cover-up.

We had resumed our surveillance duties and discovered Maria Keenahan coming out of yet another care home, Des Kelly had heard the evidence at the Ashford Tribunal and even then he still managed to go home and sleep every night, knowing that Maria Keenahan was alone with the defenceless even then BUPA refused to act and stop the abuse.

So yet again we told a horrified Dick Turner and yet again Maria Keenahan was removed from another home, in the end Dick Turner could only stop Maria Keenahan from working on his patch, BUPA refused to sack her but only agreed to move her out of their homes in this area.

They were so fiercely loyal to a known abuser that it took me years to understand, then one day some years later a reporter from the BBC rang me and said he had just interviewed BUPA's Peter Ludford, and had asked him why BUPA kept Maria Keenahan in their Employment, Mr Ludford turned to the camera and said on the record, "We did not want any one else employing her." I realised that had some one other then BUPA employed her, then BUPA's secret may have got out and they had to protect their reputation at any price but no reputation is worth the price paid by the victims.

It was now the summer of 2005 and the press had covered the latest developments in Isard House and I was about to launch the next bombardment of letters to MPs and ministers when my Mum was taken ill and admitted to hospital for tests. My mum had been in the hospital a few days when I arrived this day and saw my sister standing in the car park and even though it was pouring with rain I knew it was tears that were running down her face. My mum had cancer and it was too far gone for them to do anything, to say that we were all devastated would be an understatement, we were all so close and my Mum was the heart of the whole family, now it felt like that heart had been wrenched out.
My mum was only seventy two and I could not imagine a world without her she was my best friend. She wanted to go home. So my sister, brother and myself worked shifts and cared for her around the clock.

Suddenly the family home looked more like a hospital, a special bed, hoist and stacks of medical supplies everywhere, my poor dad seemed to fade at the same rate my mum did, it was like this terrible nightmare had suddenly descended on us all. My mum died on September 22nd 2005, six weeks after the cancer was diagnosed.

Her funeral was arranged as she would have wanted it, I sat next to my dad and we held hands all the way as we followed the white carriage and white horses that carried my mum, she had always admired those horses when she saw them and now they carried her.

My dad was sixty eight years old, he had a bad fall and died later that day, on December 22nd 2005, exactly twelve weeks to the day my mum had died.
Everything stopped of course, it's as if I had to learn to live in a new world, a world without them, it seems everything you do takes on a different significance as you think about, the last time I did so and so mum and dad were alive and well, then to top it all I ruptured my Achilles tendon badly and ended up in plaster for nearly six months and unable to walk for nearly another six months. At first I raged against the inactivity and than one day I started to write and I couldn't stop.

All the suffering I saw in Isard House was without question so fundamentally wrong that I never imagined for a moment that anyone but a abuser would defend or justify it, never would I have thought the law would excuse it and the government ignore it, I most certainly never imagined that seven years later I would still be fighting for the truth, but it is who I have had to fight that is the most shocking thing of all.

To this day BUPA continue to deny the abuse and maintain that nothing that happened in Isard House has ever caused them any concern at all. The Law that should have protected us slapped us in the face, but much worse than this it said that the abuse was alright, it excused and justified the suffering to such an extent that even the torture inflicted on Edna was not considered worthy of comment. The law acted as a shield which defended BUPA and allowed others to suffer as a direct result.

Over a thousand people sit in the House of Commons and the House of Lords, less then twelve stood up for Edna and the others.

We petitioned the Government and they like BUPA and the law before them think the suffering to be of so little consequence that it is not even worthy of a comment.

The Health Select Committees, experts and charities debate and count the victims of elder abuse presumably looking for why it happens, they need look no further than their own nose and in many cases their own conscience.

Maria Keenahan could not be alone with a defenceless elderly person for a minute without inflicting pain and for every minute she has been allowed to continue abusing, BUPA, the law and the government, have with prior knowledge and intent been her willing accomplice.

I had accepted long ago that there could be no nice neat ending, the dramatic court scene I had once imagined where justice is finally done. I now know is something that only ever happened in the movies.
But this story was much bigger for it showed what was at the heart of the system, it was not a question of how hard I had to fight to stop abuse, it was that I ever had to fight at all.

I had always joked that one day I would write it all down and now with my leg in plaster I was doing just that.
It is only now that this story is finally told that I realise why I felt so driven to write it in the first place.
This is the truth and if these words are read by another then the truth has prevailed.

The justice I had so long sought was not to be found in any court, nor was it forthcoming from any judge, but there is a higher justice when the truth prevails.

Thank you for bearing witness for Edna, Jessie, Dot, Reg, Lil, Florie, Ivy and all the others whose suffering was held so cheap, you are their justice.

Eileen Chubb

THREE

BEYOND THE FAÇADE

I see a care industry that has become big business where Multi-Nationals can make an easy profit from consumers with no rights and when things go wrong are accountable to no one. We have legislation and guidelines that are supposed to protect the elderly but which amount to no more then Tick-lists. Whistle-blowers are dammed for speaking out and betrayed by a law that feeds this conspiracy of silence.

For the elderly person abuse can mean the difference between life and death, but it can also mean the difference between a life worth living and a living hell. They are left at the mercy of a care system whose failures extend to the very heart of the establishment to such a degree even those in authority charged with protecting the elderly have themselves become active participants in their abuse.

I had my first encounter with an elderly care Charity when group counselling was arranged for us by Social Services back in 1999, the counsellor was a very nice women called Chris, who worked for the Charity Counsel and Care, Chris gave up her own time on Sundays to see us. One Sunday she said that she would not be able to continue as her boss, a man called, Les Bright had found out who our employers were and had said "We can not be seen helping these people as BUPA will not like it."

I was shocked to be told this. It was not long before I learned that, Les Bright was a close associate of Des Kelly and BUPA sponsorship was highly valued. This first encounter with elderly care charities was the first of many.

(Les Bright no longer works for Counsel and Care)

I felt I would have failed those residents in Isard House if I did not try to change things for the better, to do that I needed to know why they were wrong in the first place, I decided to start with the basics.

What I found was plenty of fancy words which amounted to excusing and justifying abuse, calling it anything other than what it is.

The Charity Action on Elder Abuse defines abuse as,

"A single or repeated act or lack of appropriate action occurring within any relationship where there is an expectation of trust, which causes harm or distress to an older person"

The words *"Any relationship"* has lumped all abuse together and whilst there maybe some common ground, abuse by relatives is a completely different problem compared with abuse by paid carers.

The words *"Where there is an expectation of trust"* This implies the victim of abuse needs to trust their abuser before it can be considered abuse, most of those I saw abused did not trust their abusers from the outset, but they were still abused. This definition also excludes all abuse by strangers.

The words *"Older person"*, what is wrong with the word old? Perhaps the fact that we find the word old so offensive we need to change it to a more attractive and politically correct, *"Older person"* is saying a lot about us as a society.

The Charity Action on Elder Abuse says
"People can be abused in different ways, these include, Physical abuse, Psychological abuse, Financial abuse, Sexual abuse and neglect."

I could not begin to list all the ways you can abuse a person for it's in as many ways as that person is capable of being hurt, in the care system it is also in as many ways as that person has needs. I have never been able to see abuse as falling under neat headings because it leads to presumptions being made, for example:

Mary is wheelchair bound and relies on staff for most of her physical needs, she calls out when she needs to go to the toilet and then sits crying in shame when no one comes. The care worker hears Mary calling but she is a power abuser and she enjoys seeing Mary suffer, the more distressed Mary becomes the more the care worker enjoys the power she has over Mary. Mary deteriates mentally and physically over a short time, she is afraid to drink anything and she dies some months later from renal failure. This whole situation was brought about because Mary needed to use the toilet and was not taken and would be considered neglect. But Mary suffered physical abuse because it resulted in bodily harm, she also suffered psychological abuse because it involved mental suffering, and if Mary had not been elderly it may have been seen in terms of manslaughter.

Jessie suffered from dementia, she was doubly incontinent and was left sitting in her own body waste day after day, and this resulted in her skin breaking down and a bedsore that went through to the bone. Jessie died a slow and painful death as a result. Maria Keenahan was a trained nurse, she knew what she inflicting on Jessie. The experts say bedsores are neglect, in terms of abuse Jessie suffered deliberate physical and psychological abuse and if she had not been old then it would be considered murder.

Annie was left lying in urine for twelve out of every twenty four hours, the acid in her urine burned her skin, a urine burn is no different from any other kind of burn, just imagine having a really bad burn and your red raw blistered skin is then subjected to scalding hot water. That is what it's like for

Beyond The Facade

Annie, her red raw skin is left in direct contact with the same substance that caused the initial burn, her eyes are watering with the pain and the only mercy is that she thinks someone will come and help her soon as due to the dementia she has forgotten no one came yesterday or the day before and the day before that. This is what is called neglect by the experts.

Action on Elder Abuse, Chief Executive, Gary Fitzgerald
"The vast majority of abuse would fall into the category of poor practice, it's about neglect, and it's about treating people with less dignity than you would other people"

"Dignity" This is the new "in" word with the experts and the Government, I can well imagine the scene, the old lady lying in the hospital bed, starving, dehydrated and with infected bed sores, she is unable to reach the food that is plonked down on the table and taken away uneaten every day. Then along comes one of the new *"Dignity Nurses"* who inquires with a cheery "How's your dignity today Mrs Smith?" and Mrs Smith says her dignity is quite well, it's the malnutrition, dehydration and infected bedsores that are killing her, "Golly Good" replies the dignity nurse who then moves on to the next bed where an old lady is dying of thirst and no longer capable of speech at all.

It all sounds a marvellous idea on paper but the

reality is very different, but the Government look like they are doing something and it deflects attention, the experts look like they have the answers to warrant the funding they have been given, the only losers really are the old people waiting for help.

Action on Elder Abuse, "Neglect includes failing to provide food, or heat or clothing, appropriate medical attention leading to bed sores, or lack of aids needed for living"

Bed sores are not brought about by a lack of medical attention, they need medical attention after they have been brought about. A bedsore can go through to the bone, they can go deeper than a knife wound, and if you stab someone with a knife the law considers it in terms of attempted murder or grievous bodily harm. But you can deliberately inflict a bed sore to the bone and your motivation for doing so will never be questioned, it's automatically presumed to be neglect, an attack on your dignity. The term neglect implies some kind of oversight, a lapse in concentration akin to forgetting to put the empty milk bottles out or post a letter. It seems to me there is one set of rules for the care system and another for the real world, for example,

A bus driver who is fully trained and licensed as competent and safe to carry public passengers, decides one day to drive his bus into a wall and people are injured and killed as a result. The driver is brought before the courts and his defence is that he had no idea that driving his bus into a wall could cause death and injury, such a defence would be laughed out of court and the driver would go to prison.

A Care worker is documented as fully trained and competent to fulfil their duty of care, this care worker dislikes a resident called Jenny, she is considered a nuisance and in need of punishment, the care worker leaves Jenny lying in bed all day and she develops a urine burn, this is deliberately ignored by the care worker and a bed sore develops which is also ignored, Jenny dies a slow and painful death from an infected bed sore. The care worker is brought before the courts and uses the same defence as the bus driver in that she was ignorant of the consequences of her actions, would the care worker also be laughed out of court and sent to prison? No because she would never be taken to court in the first place, the experts and the law say what happened to Jenny is the result of poor practice or inappropriate behaviour which are considered neglect.

The concept of premeditation or malice aforethought is not discounted after an investigation, it is never even considered in the first place.
My idea of poor practice is a bad dress rehearsal at the local amateur dramatic group.
My idea of inappropriate behaviour is picking your

nose in public or similar, it is most certainly not the criminal acts I saw committed.

You can pick up a knife and stab someone in a moment of anger, bed sores take much longer to inflict and can involve a much higher degree of wilful intent, yet the knife wound is illegal and bed sores are not. Whilst bedsores can sometimes be the result of ignorance it can not be presumed from the outset.

The Charity Action on Elder Abuse, says "Who Abuses? The abuser is usually well known to the person being abused, they may be a partner, child or relative, friend or neighbour, a paid or volunteer care worker, a health or social worker or other professional, or someone the older person is caring for"

The above has firstly lumped all abusers together and secondly has answered the question, what does an abuser do for a living? What should have been asked is what kind of person abuses in the care system and what is their motivation to abuse?

You can never understand abuse unless you understand the abuser, that so much abuse is excused or presumed to be mere neglect is hardly surprising when such ignorance exists.

I have seen four very different types of abuser and would describe them as follows,

Beyond The Facade

1. THE IGNORANCE ABUSER.

This type of abuser would have some work experience but very little effective training and of the four abuser types this abuser is the only one that could be trained not to abuse. The below example is typical of abuse committed by an ignorance abuser.

Bill is an elderly care home resident, he has Dementia so he gets disorientated at times and needs reassurance. Bill is asleep in the lounge and two care workers come to take him to the dining room for lunch. Bill can walk but he takes a long time so the staff always use a wheelchair. The two care workers do not think it worth waking Bill, and just lift him out of his chair, Bill naturally struggles and gets very agitated and the staff considers this to be aggression.
The care workers had presumed that Bill would not understand what they were doing had they tried to explain, so they never bothered. When Bill was woken from a deep sleep by two people he thought were attacking him, he did what all human beings are programmed to do, and he could not flee the danger so he fought back. The two care workers had never considered their actions from Bill's perspective and would be horrified to be told this was abuse. Then there was the matter of Bill's mobility which should have been maintained and if he subsequently developed a pressure sore as a result then in these particular circumstances it would be the result of ignorance as intent to cause

303

harm is not involved.

Mollie is a care home resident who suffers with Dementia, she needs reassurance at times and this is recorded in her care plan. Mollie is wandering the corridors crying "Where are my children? I have lost my children" she is absolutely distraught. Several residents pass by and look away unsure what to do. Molly is walking in a living nightmare, she thinks her children are small and she has lost them, imagine a young mother in your local High Street crying her children are lost, people would never just ignore her but would try and help. But because Mollies nightmare is only real to her, several staff pass and ignore her also "She gets like that sometimes" they will tell anyone who asks. Two hours earlier Mollie had nodded of after lunch and had then woken suddenly and asked the staff where her children were, this was the exact point that Mollie needed reassurance, but Mollie was ignored so thought something must have happened to her children. If the care worker had just said her children were quite safe, Mollie would be sitting in her armchair instead of walking the corridors distraught.

You can train someone that bedsores are avoidable or the importance of fluid intake or how to reassure those residents with Dementia, these are all care issues. Under no circumstances can you train someone that hitting or kicking a defenceless old women is wrong, it is not a care issue but a moral one. To stop abuse you have to

know where ignorance ends and intent begins.
Jackie was a typical Ignorance abuser.

2. THE COMPLACENCY ABUSER.

This type of abuser will usually have worked in the
care system for some time and they will have a
good knowledge of what is considered good
practice in all areas of care, if they are ever
challenged they will be able to cite good practice
and this diverts suspicion.

This type of abuser sees their victims as less than
human and views them as part of the daily grind,
just another job to be done. The motivation behind
the abuse they inflict is that the victim is in need of
punishment and that the punishment is quite
justified as the victim has made their job harder.
The victims of this abuser are perceived as
demanding or a nuisance and the abuse that is
inflicted is premeditated and intent to cause harm
is present throughout.

A complacency abuser can inflict terrible abuse
and under no circumstances can they ever be
trained not to abuse. They are always fully aware
that what they are doing is wrong but they have
the capacity to by-pass their conscience by
distancing their victims as less than human and
deserving of punishment, they distance
themselves from any feelings of guilt or remorse
and this allows them to inflict abuse such as bed

sores, urine burns, physical assaults, intimidation, withholding food and drink or using sedative drugs as a form of restraint, the below example is typical of the abuse inflicted.

Peter is an elderly care home resident, he suffers from advanced Parkinson's disease and is no longer able to walk, he has all his mental facilities and is a very intelligent cultured man who enjoys classical music, this has made him stand out from the crowd and he is noticed by a complacency abuser. Peter is considered above himself "Who does he think he is with that classical music?" is the thought that prompts this abuser to wheel Peter over to a corner of the lounge and place a radio nearby but out of his reach, the radio is then tuned to play dance music all day. Peters spirit is broken a little more each day and he eventually gives up and refuses to get out of bed in the morning and no one noticed when the abuser deliberately left his food and drink beyond his reach. Peters care plan recorded he was eating well and he was old so when he died a short while later no one really questioned it.

Nadeen was a typical complacency abuser.

3 THE POWER ABUSER.

This is the most dangerous abuser of all because of their motivation to abuse, whilst the complacency abuser can inflict similar levels of abuse whilst by-passing their conscience the power abuser has no recognisable conscience, a complacency abuser avoids the guilt of doing wrong whilst a power abuser revels in the fact it is wrong and for that reason is able to inflict suffering on a much greater scale, if abuse were seen in terms of productivity then the power abuser would always get the prize.

The power abuser will have usually worked in the care system for some time, they are there to abuse first and foremost. They need the thrill of abuse and power is their motivation for doing so, it's the thrill behind a rapist's motivation to rape which is not for any sexual gratification but for the power over another it brings.

This abuser will have an excellent knowledge of the care system and if challenged will always have a very plausible reason to explain their behaviour, they are highly intelligent and can either recite every guideline in the book on what is considered good practice, or they can just as easily play the part of the ignorance abuser, in fact they are often mistaken for just that and considered in need of training, however the reality is their knowledge would qualify them as an ideal teacher to carry out that training.

This abuser seems very ordinary, no horns protrude from their head, nor are there three sixes visible anywhere, in fact them seem very nice people and are often popular with staff and management, this is a part they play well in order to access the vulnerable, they need to seem very nice and they enjoy the challenge that is involved in appearing to be as it's all part of the game.

They are addicted to the power they obtain from inflicting suffering on others, the types of abuse that is inflicted varies from the instant gratification obtained from kicking, punching, slapping, sexual assaults and intimidation, through to the more prolonged forms of torture such as bed sores, urine burns, withholding food and drink or pain relief, through to threats of violence and isolation. One of the greatest sources of satisfaction is obtained from the victims fear of what's yet to come, even those victims with the most advanced forms of Dementia and memory loss, can retain enough recollection on some level for they can cower like frightened animals when catching sight of a power abuser.

The ultimate kicks for a power abuser is playing Russian Roulette, their power to control life and death, they can allow someone life or take it, this is done by administering potentially lethal doses of medication, the risk of discovery is only an added excitement and all part of the game as is obtaining the drugs in the quantities they need. The medication records can often be mistaken for a case of poor record keeping but the more games of Russian Roulette are played the greater the need to repeat the excitement and the more risks will be taken, the greater the risk, the greater the buzz it's the same thrill of discovery that drives the wealthy person to shoplift, it's not for the goods they steal but for the kicks.

A power abuser can only be described as pure evil and for some reason there is a refusal to believe a human being could be capable of such evil, perhaps it's a fear of confronting what we are all capable of as human beings that stops us confronting and accepting this level of pure evil, this is what allows the power abuser to abuse and is what allowed Dr Harold Shipman to kill so many, it was just easier to believe it was not happening.

The first step in stopping this abuser is to acknowledge they exist, the second step is to accept where they are likely to be found in numbers, nature tells us you will always find the predators where the prey is most plentiful.

Typical power abusers include, Maria Keenahan and Sarah Conway.

4. THE LOOK THE OTHER WAY ABUSER.

The look the other way abuser covers the largest area and contributes to more abuse than any other abuser, they know abuse is taking place and they are in a position of authority to stop it but choose not to do so. This abuser can be a care home manager, the Chief Executive of a large care company with a chain or homes, the owner of a home care agency or any other authority figure in the care system.

The initial failure to act when informed of the abuse can be for any number of reasons such as fear reputation will be damaged by allegations of abuse, or just complacency that abuse is an acceptable part of the care business and not really a problem at all.

What ever the initial motivation, the failure to act then becomes the main incentive to keep the abuse quiet which inevitably leads to more abuse being committed and which is equally denied and covered up, for to acknowledge it in any way would be to acknowledge the initial failure to act. It escalates into a vicious circle of more abuse and ever more denial.

The member of staff who reported the abuse will often be so disheartened by this failure to act, that they will leave the home and find employment in another care home or worse still they will leave the care system, yet these are exactly the very staff that should be valued by the care industry, yet what we have is a care industry that will move heaven and earth to retain the Maria Keenahan's of this world.

Another part of the ripple affect that this type of abuser causes is that the staff in a care home will be sent the wrong message, "Commit abuse but never report it."

Beyond The Facade

Typical look the other way abusers in the care system include, Val Gooding C.B.E, Des Kelly, Carole Jones, Carole Newton and Maria Green. But this type of abuser extends much further than the care system, it includes the law and the Government and even some Charities.

When I first started out I wanted to find that someone was doing something to stop abuse, I did not want to so I really wanted to find someone who was, but the more I looked the more shocked I was by what I found. I remember seeing a nice glossy BUPA care homes brochure which promised the best care, that I expected but what I did not expect was the endorsements of large Charities such as Age Concern and Help the Aged covering every page. I felt so angry that I wrote to the heads of these Charities and asked them how many inspections of the homes they carried out before endorsing them, I said their name was trusted as they were supposed to be the champions of the elderly and with that trust came a responsibility to ensure the homes they endorsed were safe, they never replied to my letters, presumably because they had never set foot in the homes they recommended.

It seemed to me that the very people who should be fighting for the elderly are not really Charities at all but part of the Corporate Business sector that profit's from elderly care.
I must have been extremely naive when I started

311

out as it never occurred to me that these Charities would take Government funding or donations from Care Companies, I do not believe that can you serve the interests of the elderly whilst in the pay of either as there is a clear conflict of interest.

Recently the large care company Southern Cross were in legal case which involved an elderly resident being asked to leave one of their care homes due to a breakdown of trust with the relatives of this person. It does not seem a big deal until you consider that it's widely accepted that moving elderly people can often result in them dying soon afterwards, and then it's more than a minor inconvenience that's involved. Which of the big Charities is fighting for the elderly person? Certainly not those Charities who took large donations from Southern Cross, perhaps the promise of future donations might deter them from coming to the aid of the elderly person in such a situation.

Perhaps you can learn to look the other way, maybe the Government could make it part of a training programme, they could call it something like, how to excuse abuse so you do not have to take any action, I shouldn't joke someone at the Health Department might take it as their latest brainwave, well it could happen when you consider their past endeavours. But on the other hand why should the Health Department bother to excuse abuse when they can pay someone else to do it for them.

Gary Fitzgerald, Action on Elder Abuse,
"The experience of the Action on Elder Abuse
help-line is that poor practice forms the greatest
percentage of abuse perpetrated by paid staff,
subsequently Action on Elder Abuse promotes
training as one guaranteed method for reducing
the potential to abuse"

You can not train most abusers and even training
the good staff would have a detrimental effect, all
good carers already know what abuse is and I
dread to think how disheartened they would feel if
Mr Fitzgerald told them what they know as abuse
is after all only poor practice. Then we have the
carers who take the risk and speak out losing their
jobs as a result, what will protect them? Certainly
not a law that leaves employers shaking with
laughter.

Mr Fitzgerald is part of the problem not the
solution.

THE GOOD CARER.

There are truly great care assistants in Care
Homes, Hospitals and Home Care, right across
this country, these carers are considered to be no
more than cleaners and are not considered worthy
to be called "Professional." If you say you are a
nurse you are given respect but say you are a

carer and you are not valued at all, yet I have seen these great carers work tirelessly above and beyond the call of duty every single day, their dedication, skills and great compassion would put to shame many of those who work in care and are afforded the title "Professional." I know how they have to battle the care system every single day to make a difference where it truly matters, at ground level, and yet they go unrecognised and un-thanked but worst of all their great capacity to care is no more visible to the experts than is the abusers capacity to abuse. I pay tribute to every single one of these carers for they make the difference between heaven and hell for the elderly they care for and I truly hope that difference will be recognised with professional status someday, in the meantime they are all that stands between the elderly and abuse, for you most certainly can not rely on the Government, the law and Mr Fitzgerald.

I have lost count of all the letters I have received from the Health Department, assuring me that the elderly will be protected by the latest piece of reactionary legislation, or the new impressive sounding guidelines that promotes good practice. If you did not know the heartbreaking reality of working in the care system, you could almost be lulled into a false sense of security. This fight has opened my eyes and once your eyes have been opened it is impossible to close them again.

What I had seen over the course of this battle

made me wonder if things had always been this bad and I had not noticed, did we always have this language of spin or did it creep up on us gradually like some kind of dry rot? One day you applied for a job and then you applied for a post. I suppose there's no real harm in dressing things up to make them sound more exciting, though personally I can not see the point of it. The real harm is when this language of spin is used to deliberately mislead or deceive then it becomes the enemy of truth or part of the abusers *"Toolkit."*

I decided to look at how care homes were inspected using the Governments protection, the best way of doing this was to cut through all the crap and see what was left, translate the language of spin and see what it amounts to if you said it in plain English.

1. Government Guideline states, No person moves into a care home without having their needs assessed and been assured they will be met.
Real Inspection Report states "Of the two files checked only one contained the care manager's assessment and the other file no assessment at all, graded as minor shortfall"

Translation. Well I have to continue inspecting so I will just pretend that all residents have had their needs assessed, it's not as if it affects the other guidelines I will be judging.

2. Government Guideline states, Residents assessed as needing short term care are helped to become independent and return home.
Real Inspection Report states: "The inspector noted some discrepancy with the numbers and categories for each client group registered this is being dealt with as a separate issue to this inspection but may on later inspections affect the grade, minor shortfall"

Translation. Residents are not in the right care setting so their needs can not be met which puts them at high risk of abuse, so we better get someone to deal with this separately and we can leave it out of a public report, the home is in breech of it's registration but it really is only a minor issue.

3. Government Guideline states. A resident's plan of care generated from a comprehensive assessment of needs is drawn up with each resident and provides the basis of the care delivered.
Real Inspection Report states "The care organisations care plan documentation in the main identifies areas required by regulation, four care plans were reviewed and contained some but not all the information, in one the resident had a pressure risk assessment which identified needs in this area however there was no care plan entry

*stating what action was being taken, neither did
The care plans reflect the continence, nutrition
needs for dementia, another care plan identified
pressure care needs but no information on health
care needs in the case of another there was no
diabetic dietary needs, grade minor shortfalls"*

Translation. The whole thing was a bloody mess
but the company had all the right forms even if a
lot of them were blank and that could have to do
with the fact the no *"Comprehensive
assessments"* had been carried out in the first
place, still it's not that important what's the worse
that can happen if you get a pressure sore or are
diabetic and given the wrong food? It's only minor
shortfalls really, not life and death issues.

*4. Government Guideline states. The home
promotes and maintains resident's health and
ensures access to health care services to meet
assessed needs.*
*Real Inspection Report states. "There is evidence
that a falls risk assessment and nutritional
screening are taking place, as is stated in the
previous standard some of the documentation is
not fully completed so do not give a full picture of
residents health care needs and do not meet with
current clinical guidelines, this is also true where
pressure risk assessments are not always
completed and reflected in care plans, this is also
true of residents with epilepsy where the home
has not detailed how they will maintain their health*

in the plan of care, all minor shortfalls"

Translation. This bloody assessment of needs not being done from the outset is affecting all the other standards, still there is some evidence of a falls risk assessment being done even if it does not include residents with epilepsy, who may well have a tendency to fall over, well I have seen worse so it's only minor really.

5. Government Guideline states. The home ensures residents receive a varied, appealing, wholesome and nutritious diet which is suited to individual assessed and recorded needs.
Real Inspection Report states" The home offers two hot meals a day, the menus viewed showed the food looked varied and nutritious with a choice of meals, the inspector was pleased to note the tables were laid nicely, minor shortfall"

Translation. A piece of paper said the food was good, so that must be true. What's the worst that can happen if someone is not assessed and needs help to eat which is not given, minor shortfall really.

6. Government Guideline states. The home ensures that residents are safeguarded from physical, financial or material, psychological or sexual abuse, neglect, discriminatory abuse or self harm, inhumane or degrading treatment, through deliberate intent, negligence or ignorance in accordance with written policies, the home has an adult protection procedure, including whistle-blowing which complies with the Public Interest Disclosure act and Department of health Guidance..

Real Inspection Report states "The home has a whistle-blowing policy and procedures for the protection of vulnerable adults, the procedures refer to local inter agency guidelines, a copy of which is available in the homes office, although the inspector was able to discuss issues with staff members, the inspector was not able to judge fully whether the staff had read and understood the homes procedures and guidelines, the homes induction and foundation training courses cover such areas as, what is abuse and what staff should do about it if they suspect abuse is occurring, however there are only a few members of staff who have undertaken this training. The manager of the home is now aware of what to do in such incidents and has made the inspectors aware of issues to enable speedy action to be taken by the authorities, minor shortfalls only"

Translation. The home has all the right bits of paper in the office, but staff do not know what they say. If a member of staff wanted to report the manager for not taking action to stop abuse then that member of staff could go to the office and ask the manager if they could check the Whistle-blowing policy to see if their identity would be protected and kept confidential if they went outside the home. This is only a minor shortfall when you consider that most of the staff have no training in abuse so would be unlikely to report it anyway. I told the manager what to do about reporting abuse as she did not know either and the manager said it was strange I should mention that as she had some abuse to report and now she could report it, so speedy action could now be taken on the abuse that was reported to her six months ago.

7. Government Guideline states, the home operates a thorough recruitment procedure based on equal opportunities and ensuring the protection of residents.
Real Inspection Report states. "Two personal files were checked from a variety of staff roles and were generally well organised, the were some gaps in the information including the required criminal records check for two non care staff, there was evidence gaps in employment had been explored, Minor shortfalls only"

Translation. It's only a minor shortfall after all criminal records checks are not important you have more chance of winning the lottery then finding an abuser with a criminal record anyway, and they were non care staff so it's not that bad, it's like expecting a school caretaker to have the same checks as teaching staff, a waste of time doing that.

Beyond The Facade

I found that regular changes were made to the inspecting of care homes, the style of the reports were changed or the name of the organisation doing the inspections was changed, for example The National Care Standards Commission changed it's name to The Commission for Social Care Inspection, all the same inspectors just carry on doing the same job in exactly the same way they always did it and it deflected attention from the latest outcry over elderly abuse, the new re-named organisation would say that was not their fault it was the people running things before us. I presume the Government think changing the name of an incompetent agency will give the public the impression something has changed.

The latest new and approved inspection reports only grade half of the guidelines that were previously thought important, I presume this is done on the basis that if you give the public only half of the information, then there will only be half of the incompetence exposed. These new reports also state what is wrong a bit more clearly but have also made it clear the usual action will be taken for non compliance, which is no action at all no matter how serious the shortfalls. Finally you now have to flick to the back of the report to find the grade awarded, In the hope you will have forgotten what appalling mess has been graded a minor shortfall by the time you find the right page.

Real Improved Inspection Report states "The residents had food stained clothing and were given very little assistance to eat despite obvious problems. One resident was served her meal later in the lounge on her own, the member of staff placed the plate of food, glass of juice on a small coffee table with only a fork to eat it, the resident was very confused and not able to feed herself, she spilt all the juice, the inspector waited a while and then attracted the attention of the member of staff, who said they were getting a knife but were observed clearing tables, this is unacceptable practice and was raised at the last inspection, when staff said they would re-heat food for residents but were observed throwing it away, grade minor shortfalls only"

Translation. So leaving residents without food and drink is considered to be *"Unacceptable practice"* but not so unacceptable as to warrant a grade of major shortfalls. If a resident is unable to feed themselves then waiting for staff to bring a knife is pretty pointless. If this is what staff are doing when inspectors are watching what the hell is happening the rest of the time? Death from malnutrition or dehydration is more then likely it's probable. So even when the evidence is there before these protectors of the elderly, nothing is done about it, not even when it was noted in a previous inspection six months earlier that uneaten food was being thrown away.

I do not think you need some kind of medical

degree to know that we die without food and drink, perhaps I should ask Bob Geldof to intervene or the Red Cross might fly in aid.

Real Inspection Report (Improved inspection of medication)"Records had been left lying about with a risk of mislaying these records, controlled drugs were checked and whilst they corresponded to the amounts recorded, there were gaps in the records including signatures and amounts received for some residents Minor shortfall.

Translation. It's always very convenient for an abuser to say they have lost the medication records especially when they are incriminating, as to the controlled drugs being checked according to what's alleged as been given, the way to check them would have been to cross reference what came into the home, only conveniently this information has gone astray also, and still all this amounts to is a minor shortfall.

Real Inspection Report (Improved inspection of medication)"The medication charts were inspected, the standard of record keeping was poor, one residents medication chart had been altered and the information changed, this chart had no record in respect of a medication that commenced in December, additionally it was evident that many morning medications had been omitted for days leaving residents at risk of not receiving medication required to maintain health, Minor shortfalls only"

Translation. Records have been fabricated and it just so happens that these records belong to a resident that has been administered drugs for six months that are not even recorded as prescribed for them, so these drugs must be obtained from illegal sources, which just might explain the drugs not given to other residents for days on end, and still only a minor shortfall to boot.

Real Inspection Report (Improved inspection of medication)"On one unit there was a duplication of medication charts, there appeared to be some confusion from the lack of signatures, handwritten transcriptions had no records of medications amounts received into the home, minor shortfall"

Translation. Double up the sheets and you can administer twice the medication, if not even an inspector can pin point what medication came in to the home, went out or was administered to the residents, than how does this protect the vulnerable? What's more it's considered yet again to be only a minor shortfall.

So this is the recently improved version of the protection, the Government say the elderly will be protected from medication abuse as G.Ps will now review the medication they prescribe to their elderly patients every six months, who will review the medication the elderly are given that is not prescribed is what I would like to know.

An abuser knows better than any care home inspector how to get round the system, the lost medication records, the handwritten prescriptions, the duplicated records, these are just a few of the numerous tactics used by abusers every day. When you cut the crap and look at what's left it is hard to believe that any one in their right mind would think it protected the elderly from abuse.

Meanwhile the trail of disasters these care homes have the cheek to call medication procedures are accepted with total complacency and graded as just *"Minor Shortfalls."* I am sure that these same Authorities if asked, would rate the lack of life boats on the Titanic as a minor shortfall, as long as The White Star Line had all the right policies and procedures in their office, but policies and procedures are no use when you are drowning.

The elderly victims of abuse are not able to vote, they are not able to take to the streets in protest, if they could then the Government would have taken effective action long ago, it seems their lives are not worth care home inspections that actually protect them, we have a care industry calling for less regulation and scrutiny and a Government all too willing to oblige.

Eileen Chubb

No one uses this new language of spin more than the Government, who would not dare tell you anything in plain English, presumably because they are too ashamed of it. After all, the recent public outcry over abuse in care homes, this is what the Government thinks will stop abuse.

Inspecting for better lives is the name of the latest Government brain wave, the first thing that struck me was that the term elderly in need of care seems to be avoided at all costs, the reasoning being that if you play down the vulnerability then the protection will look more effective. So the preferred word is *"Service user."* This term conjures up the image of an elderly lady who is totally independent and needs no care, who is out with her shopping trolley looking for a bargain in the *"Care packages"* section of the local super market. The real *"Service user"* is more likely to be totally dependent on the care of others and who is unable to participate in *"Public consultations"* due to Dementia or other illness. If this real person was asked to choose between a fancy title or being safe they would chose being safe, the term *"Service user"* does not empower, it hides how much the vulnerable are at risk.

The next word in this dictionary of spin is *"Stakeholder"* which apparently is not a job description for an assistant vampire slayer, but a term often used in public consultations so that who was consulted about what is not very clear, for example you could have different groups of people being consulted about something in a care home, the residents, the staff and the company who own the home and a charity representing the elderly, who is sponsored by the company who own the home, so a "*Stakeholder*" is someone with a vested interest but not necessarily without a conflict of interest.

The new allegedly improved inspection reports were one of the suggested improvements that came from a Government public consultation document entitled *"Inspecting for better lives"* given it's contents it would have better suited the title, *"Inspecting for an easy life."* The following extracts are taken from this document and under each extract a translation into English was required.

SPIN. "Individuals who use or receive regulated services engaged through the Quality work shops and interviews facilitated by OPM"

Translation, we asked the people who received care what they wanted, we paid a public consultation company to gather this information, leaving aside the fact it is information obtained from people who are often unable to communicate, which is why they have care needs in the first place. We are not stating how many of these people suffered from Dementia or were physically totally dependant as that would make the whole "*Quality workshop interviews*" thing look a bit stupid.

SPIN. "Developing a provider quality assessment self assessment, that has the experiences of the people using the services at its core"

Translation. We do not know how to ask the people using the services that have already allegedly been consulted without them getting wind of what we are up to, and we do not know how to design the new tick list, which the care home will use to grade itself after it has inspected itself. The problem is we do not know how to include the experiences of the residents in the home, as firstly most of them would not be in the home if they were able to *"Relate their experiences"* and secondly the police might be called if they did so.

SPIN. "Some providers with well developed quality assurance systems offered to help us developing this component of the new approach, which we will take up"

Translation. Because we do not know how to make the tick lists, the big Care Companies have very kindly offered to design the tick lists they will use to grade themselves, which we are happy to let them do as they have much more experience at making bit's of paper look impressive enough to pass for good care.

SPIN."A theme of concern running through the response was the challenge to our work force of an approach which has concentrated on processes to one which focuses on results for people using services, the need for on going work force development and good quality assurance systems was emphasised in many of the letters we received"

Translation. They think we are crap at our job and always have been and can not see any reason why we will not continue to be crap. Bloody people writing in with letters can not be controlled like those who filled in our Questionnaire.

To summarise, there is a huge public outcry when it is estimated that up to half a million elderly people are being abused at any one time, the Governments response is not to stop the abuse, but to stop the public outcry over it, a stance that amounts to "We can not have all this abuse being reported, we need to stop looking for it."
 So all the good care homes *(The ones with only minor shortfalls)* can inspect themselves and then the Government can claim credit for the massive improvement (According to their reliable figures) in care home standards that will inevitably result, well on paper anyway. The are many words that sum this up but the waste product of a male bovine immediately springs to mind.

Eileen Chubb

Imagine if Restaurants or Hotels started awarding themselves stars, the whole star rating system would lose all credibility over night, the very idea is so ridiculous it would never even be contemplated in the first place, yet that is exactly what is proposed for care homes, but what is even more ridiculous is they expect people to believe their spin. The worst thing that can happen if a Restaurant over rates itself is the food will be a disappointment, allow care homes to do this and it is people's lives that are put at risk.

The Governments reaction to elder abuse amounts to a tick list heaven for the care industry, a behind closed doors strategy that adds to the silence that already allows abuse to thrive.

I do not understand how you can look away, how do you convince yourself it is not really happening because it all looks good on paper, I do not have that luxury and God knows I want an easy life as much as the next person, but I can still hear the screams and remember the pain and I know that right now elderly people are being abused and their only hope is someone will hear their screams or notice their bruised bodies, and this is happening whilst the Government turns a blind eye to human rights abuses it would most certainly condemn were they taking place in any other country.

So the Government do nothing, the experts continue to count the victims of abuse and people like Edna wait for the day when the magic number is reached, when finally enough people have suffered to warrant action, meanwhile the law continues to fail those who need it's protection the most and shields abusers to such a degree that it becomes no law at all but an accomplice in the crime.

Who of these is the guiltier?

The power abuse that inflicts unimaginable torture and suffering every single day she works with the defenceless?

The care home inspector, who knows people are being abused, justifies it as a minor shortfall and walks away?

The expert from Action On Elder Abuse, Mr Fitzgerald, who described the force feeding of talcum powder as "*Teasing*" and calls what are torture regimes, "*Poor practice*"?

The Judge who found an excuse to make kicking a defenceless old women alright?

The Care Company who crucifies Whistle-blowers whilst the law looks on?

The man who sits in 10 Downing Street, knows abuse is happening, has the power to stop it, but looks the other way rather than upset the powerful care home industry?

None is the guiltier that are all equally guilty.

I went to the Relatives and Residents Association annual conference a few years ago, my dear friend and fellow campaigner, Gillian Ward got us tickets. We were unfamiliar with the local area and got a little lost which meant we arrived just in time to find a seat at the back of the hall before the conference began. It was all very impressive and all the respected experts who had been invited clapped loudly as each of the speakers in turn said elder abuse was not to be tolerated and that it would be stopped.

When we broke for lunch I caught sight of a man at the front who had just turned toward me, it was Des Kelly, my heart was racing as I turned to Gillian and told her who was there, Gillian knew all about our case so knew who Des Kelly was by name and she went as pale as me as we made our way to the room where lunch was being served. I saw Des Kelly and Les Bright sitting together a little way off, birds of a feather I thought.

The afternoon speaker was to be Paul Burstow M.P who I knew well as he is one of the few who have actually done something about abuse. They said when Mr Burstow had finished speaking that we could ask questions and there was a girl in the aisle that would bring a microphone to anyone with a question. I snatched the microphone and without even looking at Paul Burstow I said "There are some people who talk the talk but do not walk the walk and one such person is in this room today"

I pointed at Des Kelly and heard chairs scrape back as several people stood to get a better look at the man I pointed at, there was this deathly silence in the room and I just found the words coming out of my mouth, "That man sits there under a cloak of respectability, the same man I went to for help, the same man who denied and covered up abuse and stood by whilst the Whistle-blowers who reported it, went in fear for their own safety, well he stood on the wrong side when it mattered most and he has not a shred of decency or shame and he makes me sick."

I than looked down at the microphone and up at Paul Burstow and remembered I was supposed to be asking him a question, so I said as an afterthought, "Do you think Whistle-blowers should be better protected?" There was a stunned silence and than Paul Burstow said "Yes" and then he launched into how he had seen me on the Television last week and he agreed with everything I had said about it.

I could hardly believe that I had stood up in a conference room full of people and said what needed to be said. Des Kelly sat through the rest of the conference with his head down. Just before I left a man in the hallway said to me, "Do you know who Mr Kelly is?" I of course knew Des Kelly was a respected expert in the circles that attend Charity conferences and such like, I looked the man straight in the eye and said "Oh yes I know who Mr Kelly is but more importantly I know what he is."

I dare say I left a few wagging tongues in my wake that day but I hope I also opened a few eyes to the hypocrisy that exists.

So what hope for those like Edna and Jessie who wait for someone to stop their suffering right now, their only hope is a Whistle-blower.

WHISTLE-BLOWING.

Every day Mr Smith makes the same Train journey to and from work, he boards the Train, and reads his Newspaper, he never considers the possibility that he may never get off that Train again, of course in the back of his mind he knows that Trains can crash, but that kind of thing happens to other people, not to him. When Mr Smith boards his train every day he entrusts his life to a Train Company he knows nothing about.

Jack works for the Train Company, it is his job to inspect the tracks, one day Jack discovers the tracks in a certain section are in a dangerous state, he reports this immediately to his manager. Jack knows that there could be an accident at any time and he tells his manager that the section should be closed down for urgent repairs. But the section is on a very profitable route so the Train Company decide a weekend repair schedule will do. Jack knows that it is too dangerous to allow Trains to continue to run. He also knows that if he blows the whistle to the Authorities he would be risking his job.

Jack desperately needs his job, he has a mortgage and a young family to support, most people will say that Jack should blow the whistle and risk all, we expect a lot from those who are in Jacks position, and so should we not expect the law to protect Jack if he speaks out? What if jack was not willing to risk his job, what if Jack had seen a workmate sacked for whistle-blowing, what if Jack did not trust the law, should we trust our life to what if?

Fine words are said about *"Open Government"* but not too open it seems as The Freedom of Information Act has been considered too free. The Public Interest Disclosure Act has now been considered too public and a behind closed doors policy of mediation has been enforced; actions speak louder than words.

I admit that I am very protective of Whistle-blowers, how could I not be when I have seen first hand what happens to them. If anyone thinks that the current law protects them, then I sincerely hope that they never have to blow the whistle, but most of all I hope their life never depends on someone else doing so.

God knows if the law offered a scrap of protection I would have found it by now, the law is one thing, the reality is something entirely different.

THE LAW encourages disclosures be made to the employer first.

THE REALITY.

Sharon works in the Accounts Department and she discovers that the Company is fiddling its workers pension fund, she reports this to her boss, but he is involved in the fiddling so he takes no action.

Sharon could go to the Authorities, but the Company would know it was her as she already reported this to her boss. She is frightened she will lose her job, she wishes she had not told her boss first. The law has firstly put Sharon at risk and secondly made it more likely that the crime will not be reported.

THE LAW allows for disclosures to be made to an outside Authority first but there are more stringent requirements to be met.

THE REALITY.

Sharon decides to look at the Company Whistle-blowing Policy, it states she should report concerns to her line manager and then his line manager and so on but they are involved in the fiddling so she can not do that, the policy states she can report it outside the company to the relevant authority and that her identify would be protected. But her boss would know it was her because she was the only person who had access to the accounts other those involved in the fiddling, and if she went to the Authorities she would have to report her boss for not acting. The conduct of Sharon's boss has now been called into question, which becomes a disclosure of wrong-doing in itself, this can only lead to a "Them or me" situation, where the boss denies he was informed and tries to discredit Sharon and/or denies any wrong doing has taken place and attempts to cover-up or destroy any evidence to the contrary. Sharon is then left at the mercy of a boss who has every incentive to harass her. The laws requirements have directly brought about a situation where harassment, wrong-doing going unreported or a cover-up is more likely to take place.

Sharon is prepared to risk her job and reports the fraud, whilst her allegations are being investigated she is harassed by her employer and made ill she takes sick leave and resigns a while later, she takes her case to an Employment Tribunal claiming constructive dismissal as a result of making protected disclosures, if she had not reported the fraud she would still have had her job.

Sharon's boss uses the defence of absolute denial in that Sharon was not harassed and that the fraud did not take place. The Employment Tribunal then have to judge if there was harassment and they also have to judge if there was fraud, Given that serious concerns have been raised about a jury's ability to understand complicated fraud cases, it is incredible that no one bats an eye at an Employment Tribunal judging such matters.

THE LAW separates the Whistle-blower from the disclosures.

THE REALITY.

Jean works in a care home and sees elderly people being abused. Jean clearly considers this to be wrong and reports the abuse to her manager with the expectation the manager will view it as equally wrong. The manager fails to take any action, it is from this point on that the law should not separate the Whistle-blower from the disclosures, because once the manager failed to act Jean suffered a loss or detriment as the law refers to it.

Jean cared enough to make the disclosures of abuse to her manager, when nothing was done to stop the abuse, then Jean lost all trust. Jean felt she had two choices, firstly she could leave and work elsewhere or she could report the abuse to the authorities and hope she did not lose her job, either way Jeans job was lost because the manager did not act.

Most cases will not overcome the huge odds that are stacked against them and will never make it as far as an Employment Tribunal, the only hope of protection is from the few cases that do make it, that those who have been genuinely victimised will be protected by the law, sending out a strong message that harassment of Whistle-blowers will not be tolerated, the reality is that the opposite message is being sent. All the employer has to do is deny everything and the law will work to his benefit, the law values denial above telling the truth.

Often it is the Whistle-blower who will find he has become a problem and not the wrongdoing he reported.

John has worked for a Finance Company for over fifteen years and has an exemplarily work record and considered to be very good at his job. John than discovers fraud has taken place and he reports this to his boss, his boss fails to act so John reports it to the relevant Authorities. All of a sudden notes are being made on Johns staff file which state that his work is substandard, the tasks that he once carried out daily and was commended for, are now being criticised. John is eventually placed under supervision and the criticism mounts, John knows it is only a matter of time before enough evidence has been fabricated against him for him to be dismissed from his job and he worries how this would look on his work record. Every day that John goes to work it become harder to bear and finally one day the strain becomes too much and he takes sick leave. This is where John should be able to claim the protection of the law.

The law that said to the BUPA seven they were off sick so were not subjected to any detriment. (File notes commending their work record showed that criticism of their work commenced on the day they blew the whistle) The employers conduct in falsifying documentation is not worthy of comment. The law sees no connection to reporting abuse and being made ill, the law sees no detriment in loss of salary.

The Hospital manager (Ian Perkins) who had an exemplarily work record before he blew the whistle on dishonesty, found to his dismay that his work was no longer commendable but just the opposite in fact and he was sacked for his attitude. The law said that he had defended himself too robustly at his disciplinary hearing, by calling numerous colleagues to vouch for him, the law said this was the attitude that led to him being sacked, the evidence of all the independent witness's which was submitted to the Tribunal and contradicted his employers assertions were discounted.

The Nurse who discovered that a child had a "Do not resuscitate" order placed on her without the knowledge of the parents, the nurse informed the parents and was then so severely harassed she was forced to take sick leave, the law held her subsequent dismissal to be lawful as she was sacked for being sick and not for blowing the whistle and the law could see no connection between the two.

The law not only failed to protect these Whistle-blowers it slapped them in the face for good measure, for every case that makes it as far as a Tribunal there are hundreds that could not overcome the insurmountable barriers that are placed in their path, for the few that do make it at the cost of terrible hardship, such verdicts are a crime against justice.

When Employment Tribunals or Industrial Tribunals as they were called, were first established the aims were to reduce pressure on the civil courts and give quick and easy access to a legal remedy in a setting where both employers and employees could represent themselves. Things have drastically changed over the years and most cases now involve Barristers and Solicitors, this has hugely tipped the scales of justice in favour of the Employer, who could be a Multi National Company for example and have the unlimited financial might to access the very best legal representation that money can buy.

The worker on the other hand has to fend for himself as there is no legal aid available to bring a case in an Employment Tribunal, not even for cases that are in the public interest to be heard.

The Whistle-blower is expected to either save up before reporting any abuse or obtain legal representation on a, "No win, No fee" arrangement. Such arrangements incur a serious conflict of interest. A solicitor can have their fees guaranteed by the other side on condition they advise their clients to settle out of court. This means that in Public Interest Disclosures Cases, evidence that has been disclosed will never be made public. In such a situation would the advice of a solicitor be in the client's interests or the solicitors interests? The fact that such a question arises in the first place is not in the interests of justice, in any type of legal case, but in Public Interest Disclosure cases it is a parody of justice, as the law that allegedly upholds the public interest actually harms it instead.

Recent changes in Tribunal rules now make it nearly impossible to have your day in court. The workers rights are forfeit if they do not enter into mediation with their employer, prior to taking their case to a Tribunal. This mediation amounts to negotiation and out of court settlements are being encouraged, so the disclosures in the public interest will be even less likely to be made public.

The law fails again to recognise the importance of the disclosures to the Whistle-blower and the irretrievable loss of trust in the employer who failed to act on them. Mediation could never restore this trust so really it is just about the employer trying to buy silence, why should the worker forfeit his rights for not selling his soul.

What the law expects from the worker.
The full burden of proof is placed on the worker, which requires a much greater degree of legal input from the party who is more likely to have very limited legal resources if indeed any at all. This can hardly be considered a level playing field.

What the law accepts from the employer.
An Employer who took no action to rectify a situation that led to a worker losing his job and taking a case to a Tribunal, will often submit evidence to that Tribunal of what steps he took after the worker obtained a solicitor. In summary once the damage is done to the worker the employer will often remember his duty of care and submit letters between solicitors in support of this, not only is such evidence admissible but it is actually relied upon in verdicts that find for the employer.
For example I tell two senior BUPA managers we are being harassed, they do nothing so we are forced out of our jobs, six months later once we have a solicitor, BUPA say they are willing to put

up a notice on the staff notice board in all homes saying harassment is not allowed. This letter offering to take any kind of action after we had resigned is considered evidence in their defence.

When the Employer totally denies any abuse has taken place, if that abuse is subsequently upheld to be true, than it should detract from the employers credibility when it came to judging the harassment, which is equally denied. The Tribunal will however disregard the evidence of the relevant authority and proceed to judge the disclosures.

The first problem with this is that disclosures are likely to relate to criminal offences and an Employment Tribunal has no qualifications, experience or even jurisdiction to judge criminal acts.

Secondly I see no point in placing a burden on the worker to report to the correct Authority, if the conclusions of that authority are ignored, if the law can not even accept the evidence of the very authority it required the worker to disclose to, than the law fails to protect the disclosures, never mind the whistle-blower.

Absolute denial is such an effective defence because we have a law that actively encourages and rewards the culture of Cover-up, never hands-up, and the very culture that led to the need for the whistle-blowing in the first place.

Beyond The Facade

The Government says the law aims to encourage employers to develop whistle-blowing policies which will protect whistle-blowers, but policies and procedures are just bit's of paper at the end of the day, when I was in Isard House I could have gone to the homes office and taken the numerous policies and procedures and stuffed them down my clothing as padding, so when I was hit in the back with a chair they would have offered some protection as body armour, but that is the extent of the protection they offered.

What makes a law work is enforcement, there is not a policy and procedure in the world that alone would stop someone breaking the law. To expect it is like saying murder is illegal but you will not be punished if you commit it. If something is against the law than it is up to the law to send out a strong message that it will not be tolerated. A law that will not stand up in court is worse then no law at all. It gives people who need the protection false hope and it becomes a joke to those who break it. There is no incentive for employers to comply with the law, the chances are the truth will never come out in court.

There are many injustices in the legal system and we are all too familiar with the stories of people who have been wrongly imprisoned, it is small wonder to me that the justice system fails those accused of doing wrong when it can not even protect those who have done right.

Eileen Chubb

THE SHIPMAN INQUIRY. CHAPTER ELEVEN.

Raising concerns.

Page 337. Evidence from Dr Ian Hargraves.
"It may well be that the perception at the front line is that policies and procedures are regarded as fine words, which do not reflect the approach that will be taken in practice"

Page 328. On the evidence of Mr Guy Dehn.
Public Concern at Work.
(The man who wrote the Public Interest Disclosure Act)
Dame Janet Smith says "Mr Dehn was at pains to emphasise however that neither the number of Employment Tribunal decisions nor the sums awarded are the correct measures of the success of The Public Interest Disclosure Act, the primary purpose of which was to create a culture where employees could report concerns"

BUPA has a culture where you can report concerns; it is what happens to you afterwards that is the problem.

I am not surprised that Mr Dehn was at pains to emphasise his act should not be measured in the court room. It is the last place it could be used effectively.

I know that The Public Interest Disclosure Act fails

to protect Whistle-blowers, it amounts to a lot of
fine words that sound very impressive until you
live the reality of claiming it's protection, it is just
another piece of paper written by another
esteemed expert who has no idea what it's like to
be spat at, assaulted and threatened day after day
until you can not take it anymore, the law says it
will not stand idly by, well the law did exactly that.

It has been a long hard fight but I would do it all
again without a second's hesitation, it has cost me
a great deal in so many ways but it would have
cost me more to look the other way.
Most of us probably tell ourselves when we see
something unjust that one person can not do
anything to change things for the better, perhaps
that is so and perhaps defeated by the law and the
system I should have given up, but the memory of
a tortured and broken human being reaching out
her hand to me is not a memory so easily erased,
I am reminded that what I am fighting for is right
and you would be amazed where the strength
comes from when right is on your side.

How can abuse be stopped?

Put as much effort into action as is currently put
into fine words, prosecute abusers and care
companies and give the elderly the same
protection as everyone else by actually applying
the laws that already exist.

Stop describing elderly abuse in the insipid social

worker spin, which makes it sound like some kind of unpleasant inconvenience.

When relatives raise concerns give them someone to go to that will actually take action instead of making excuses.

Stop making documentaries about yet another under-cover reporter who is shocked by the abuse he films, it's time to move beyond that, it's turned into a standard entertainment format to film abuse. Start making documentaries about what the law did to the criminals involved in the crimes. It may give the law some incentive to do something for a change.

Recognise and reward with professional status good carers and make elderly care a profession in its own right, with its own professional conduct committee that actually punishes misconduct.

Protect Whistle-blowers who speak out with a law that calls to account employers who value their reputations above those in their care.

Stop giving honours to the likes of Des Kelly and Val Gooding, who have been amply paid for their " Services to the care industry"

Look at how much profit is being made by these big companys before accepting their excuses about abuse being the result of lack of public investment.

Beyond The Facade

The only way to build a care system that's fit to care is to strip away the façade and start again.

When I needed someone to help me stop Maria Keenahan torturing anymore defenceless people, it should have been the police, the council and the law that should have come to my aide but it was the press, I would especially like to thank,

Heather Mills (No relation to Mills McCartney), and everyone at Private Eye, a true champion of truth and justice.

Lucy Johnston.

Jamie McGinnis.

Richard Simcox.

Jenny Chyrss.

Sam Hart.

Eileen Chubb

INDEX

Private Eye 4/3/05, BUPA DON'T CARE HOMES.
By Heather Mills.

Former care staff who made serious allegations of
neglect, potentially fatal doping and mistreatment
of old people at Isard House, a BUPA run care
home near Bromley in Kent, have at last learned
what action police took in response to a dossier of
evidence they submitted three years ago, it was all
but ignored.

No statement was taken from any witness, no
member of staff from the home was interviewed
and BUPA it's self was never even approached
over the allegations. In fact police notes suggest
that just a few hours after three bundles of
documents, mainly complex medical records were
submitted officers had already decided that "No
crime had been confirmed."

This is alarming since on face value the medical
sheets seemed to show that a number of elderly
residents were given potentially fatal doses of
powerful drugs. One resident E.P (Edna) had on
four occasions been given a dose of tranquilliser
that was Nine times the daily prescribed dose,
30mls and Six times higher then what is
considered safe for an elderly person. Eye readers
may also recall the case of Audrey Ford another
Isard House resident who was taken to hospital

suffering from the side-effects of a powerful Anti psychotic which should only have been given to those suffering severe mental illness, like Schizophrenia. She never recovered and the Coroner recorded an open verdict.

The care staff have been trying for some time now to discover what progress the Police had made in there investigations and under The Freedom Of Information Act, they found out last month. A Police summery said it had decided to make only limited inquiries into the allegations. "To prevent unnecessary use of Police time for an inquiry that was unlikely to be brought before a court." Officers obtained a brief report from the Coroners office listing "Those deaths of occupants from Isard house with cause", however it said none were the subject of an inquest and the examining doctor had issued death certificates in all cases, "Therefore it must be assumed that no suspicious circumstances were identified "these were exactly the sort of assumptions the, Shipman Inquiry, condemned so vigorously.
The Police report said "As indicated only limited inquiries have been made, no persons accused have ever been interviewed, nor have BUPA been formally approached by Police to assist in the inquiry, subject to Crown Prosecution Advice, no further action will be taken "Eileen Chubb, one of the care workers, who now runs the Charity Compassion In Care, said "The Need for a public inquiry is now overwhelming, how can the crown Prosecution Service decide whether there is a

case, if the Police don't bother to investigate and gather the evidence in the first place?"

SUBMISSION EXTRACTS.

"At paragraph 31 of her statement to the Tribunal Eileen Chubb referred to the treatment of E.P (Edna) with excessive amounts of Chlorpromazine, at b4 an examination of the relevant sheets demonstrates such overdosing was being carried out"

"The Tribunal is also asked to note at 33, the label dated April 21st 1999 prescribing four to 6mls of chlorpromazine is stuck over the label at 32, prescribing 4mls, the Tribunal is asked to note that this was likely to have been done on the day that Social Services entered the home to begin it's investigation, which was on April 21st 1999 and it is submitted that a reasonable interpretation of the act of sticking a label dated April 21st over the previous label is to hide the repeated unauthorised overdosing of Chlorpromazine, when confronted with this evidence, Maria Keenahan sought to argue it away by suggesting she was merely carrying out the instructions given on the previous months sheet, when the previous months sheets were examined (p31b3) the label for dosage was missing altogether, furthermore when asked Maria Keenahan was not sure what the doses on the missing label were likely to have been and made a number of suggestions including lower then those *recorded as given"*

"It is in the area of administration of medication that objective evidence on which the reasonable beliefs to the malpractice is clearest, the Tribunal is also referred to the notes of the investigation interview held with Maria Keenahan, by Des Kelly on August 10th 1999, in which she indicates she was judging what Chlorpromazine to give"

"The Tribunal is also referred to the evidence of Amanda Chumley given during the Social Services investigation, which corroborates 31 of Eileen Chubb's statement on the earlier overdosing of chlorpromazine by Maria Keenahan. Administration of drugs in excess of prescribed levels was carried out knowingly by Maria Keenahan, further Eileen Chubb's concerns about the state of the medication has been bourn out by the report of the independent pharmacists (b4348) which was undertaken as part of the Social Services investigation, the Tribunal is particularly directed to the findings in that report in respect of EP (Edna) Further the Tribunal is invited to draw the co conclusion on the basis of the report that there were serious failings in the system of administration of medication and that the applicants that made complaints about it had good reason to do so, these include the overdosing of EP (Edna) by Maria Keenahan and a proper examination of the medication records at the time would have revealed the failings"

"In addition to Carole Jones inadequate investigation of medication, the respondents BUPA subsequent investigation carried out by Susan Greenwood, was equally inadequate, it was not until a independent survey was carried out that the serious extent of the failings became clear, such an inadequate response by BUPA to such serious complaints can only be taken as a deliberate failure to act, had the issues been taken seriously with the resources they have, BUPA could equally have obtained expert advice in the same way that Social Services did once matters were formally raised by the applicants"

Lightning Source UK Ltd.
Milton Keynes UK
UKOW040116011112

201490UK00001B/7/P